## The Pocket Guide to

# Lymphoma Classification

David Mason and Kevin Gatter

Department of Cell... University of Oxford,
John Radcliffe Hosp...

D1099420

**Blackwell**

© 1998 by
Blackwell Science Ltd
Editorial Offices:
Osney Mead, Oxford OX2 0EL
25 John Street, London WC1N 2BL
23 Ainslie Place, Edinburgh EH3 6AJ
350 Main Street, Malden
    MA 02148 5018, USA
54 University Street, Carlton
    Victoria 3053, Australia
10, rue Casimir Delavigne
    75006 Paris, France

Other Editorial Offices:
Blackwell Wissenschafts-Verlag GmbH
Kurfürstendamm 57
10707 Berlin, Germany

Blackwell Science KK
MG Kodenmacho Building
7–10 Kodenmacho Nihombashi
Chuo-ku, Tokyo 104, Japan

First published 1998

Set at the Medical Informatics Unit
Department of Cellular Science
University of Oxford
Printed and bound in Italy
by Vincenzo Bona s.r.l., Turin

DISTRIBUTORS

    Marston Book Services Ltd
    PO Box 269
    Abingdon, Oxon OX14 4YN
    (*Orders*: Tel: 01235 465500
            Fax: 01235 465555)

USA
    Blackwell Science, Inc.
    Commerce Place
    350 Main Street
    Malden, MA 02148 5018
    (*Orders*: Tel: 800 759 6102
                781 388 8250
            Fax: 781 388 8255)

Canada
    Login Brothers Book Company
    324 Saulteaux Crescent
    Winnipeg, Manitoba R3J 3T2
    (*Orders*: Tel: 204 224-4068)

Australia
    Blackwell Science Pty Ltd
    54 University Street
    Carlton, Victoria 3053
    (*Orders*: Tel: 3 9347 0300
            Fax: 3 9347 5001)

A catalogue record for this title is
available from the British Library

ISBN 0-632-05096-9

# Contents

The University of Oxford Department of Cellular Science produces a number of publications for training, teaching and reference.

Publications include reference books and slide sets, which are suitable for students and professionals primarily in the fields of pathology, haematology and oncology.

Details of publications are available either from the Department or via the internet:

Department of Cellular Science
Room 5501
John Radcliffe Hospital
Headington
OXFORD
OX3 9DU
United Kingdom


Telephone: +44 (0)1865 220545
Fax: +44 (0) 1865 221693
Internet: http://phoenix.jr2.ox.ac.uk
Email: miu@cellsci.ox.ac.uk

We are grateful to Dr. Nancy Harris, Prof. Peter Isaacson, Dr. Elaine Jaffe and Prof. Harald Stein for helpful comments and the provision of illustrations; to Beata Ozieblowska and Bridget Watson for their patience and care in compiling the text; and to Ellie Parker for the Pocket Book design.

> "The urge to classify is a fundamental human instinct; like a predisposition to sin, it accompanies us into the world at birth and stays with us to the end."
>
> Hopwood A.T.
> *Proceedings of the Linnean Society of London*
> (1957) 171: 230–234.

Before considering previous attempts to classify lymphoid neoplasms, it is worth reflecting that the tendency to categorize is a strong human instinct. "Splitters" are often more insistent than "lumpers" so that pathologists tend to err on the side of over-classifying rather than the reverse.

**Rappaport - 1966**
**BNLI - 1973**
**Kiel / Lennert - 1974**
**Lukes / Collins - 1974**
**W.H.O. - 1976**
**Working Formulation - 1982**

Rappaport's simple classification of lymphoma was widely adopted by pathologists and clinicians but became increasingly unwieldy as it was modified to incorporate new knowledge of different lymphoma entities.

A number of more complex schemes in the 1970s attempted a fresh approach. The most widely used were those proposed by Lukes and Collins, and by Lennert and the Kiel group, but they showed little correlation with each other or with other schemes.

This was a source of considerable frustration to outsiders, as eloquently expressed in a letter by Humphrey Kay to the *Lancet*.

---

Sir - The announcement in the *Lancet* of two more classifications of non-Hodgkin's lymphomas encourages me to put forward my classification of these classifications:

Well-defined, high grade, oligosyllabic

Poorly differentiated, polysyllabic ⎯⎯⎯⎯⎯
- diffuse
- circumlocutory
- with dyslexogenesis

Unicentric ⎯⎯⎯⎯⎯
- derivative
- neologistic

Multicentric, cycnophilic
(Gk. κυκνοζ = Swan)

Cleaved and convoluted types ⎯|
- Rappaport (non-Lukes)
- Lukes (non-Rappaport)

This system makes no claim to be comprehensive or even comprehensible, so there may well be scope for other classifications of classifications and ultimately, one hopes a classification of classifications of classifications. At that point we shall need a conference in the Caribbean.

H.E.M. Kay. Royal Marsden Hospital.
The *Lancet* (1974) ii:586

---

An equally telling comment came from an American oncologist, which made, despite its facetious tone, two important points, both of which are valid today. Firstly, the separation of lymphomas into several broad categories is a reminder that oncologists require from the pathologist some indication of clinical behavior. Secondly, the fantastical names indicate that the titles given to lymphoma subtypes by pathologists often appear to be unnecessarily complex and confusing.

# Classification Schemes for Lymphoma

To the Editor: It is becoming more difficult to understand pathologists when they talk about the malignant lymphomas. Therefore, I have devised a practical classification designed to supersede the systems now commonly used. It has the advantage of being precise, predictive and relatively simple to apply.

I. Good ones (includes nonconvoluted diffuse centrilobulated histoblastoma, immune binucleolar hyperbolic folliculated macrolymphosarcoma, T2-terminal transferase-negative bimodal prolymphoblastic leukosarcoma, Jergen-Kreuzart-Munier-Abdullah syndrome and reticulated histoblastic pseudo-Sézary IgM-secreting folliculoma).

Characteristic: Small tumor that does not recur after treatment.

II. Not-so-good ones (formerly "hairy cell" pseudoincestuoblastoma, quasiconvoluted binucleate germinoma, sarcoblastiocytoma, Syrian variant of heavy-chain disease and German grossobeseioma).

Characteristic: Such tumors disappear on treatment but return and cause appreciable mortality.

III. Really bad ones (include farsical mononuclear diffuse convoluted pseudoquasihistiolymphosarcomyeloblastoma, IgG variant of fragmented plasmatic gammopathy, triconvoluted ipsilateral rhomboid fever, Armour's hyperthermic caninoma and Hohner's harmonica).

Characteristic: Regardless of treatment, such tumors keep growing.

IV. Ones that are not what they seem (include gallbladder disease, appendicitis, shotgun wounds and ingrown toenails).

Characteristic: These conditions are not actually lymphomas but are included for the sake of completeness.

Donald J. Higby, M.D Roswell Park Memorial Institute
*New England Journal of Medicine* (1979) 300:1283

| Working Formulation categories of non-Hodgkin's lymphoma |
| --- |

**Low grade**
A.   Small lymphocytic.
B.   Follicular, predominantly
          small cleaved cell
C.   Follicular, mixed
          small cleaved and large cell

**Intermediate**
D.   Follicular, predominantly
          large cell
E.   Diffuse, small cleaved cell
F.   Diffuse, mixed small and
          large cell
G.   Diffuse, large cell

**High grade**
H.   Large cell, immunoblastic
I.   Lymphoblastic
J.   Small non-cleaved cell

*Cancer* (1982) 49:2112–2135

An international nomenclature project in the late 1970s attempted to clarify matters by creating a common language for the entities in the different schemes. This new terminology, known as the "Working Formulation", was adopted by many pathologists and clinicians. However, it failed to achieve its aim of creating an international "lymphoma Esperanto", mainly because entities in one scheme did not always appear in other schemes, and *vice versa*.

### Kiel Classification of non-Hodgkin's Lymphoma

**Low grade B**
Lymphocytic - CLL, PLL, HCL
Lymphoplasmacytic / cytoid
Plasmacytic
Centroblastic / centrocytic
Centrocytic

**High grade B**
Centroblastic
Immunoblastic
Burkitt's lymphoma
Large cell anaplastic
Lymphoblastic

**Low grade T**
Lymphocytic - CLL and PLL
Small cerebriform cell (mycosis
    fungoides, Sézary syndrome)
Lymphoepithelioid (Lennert's)
Angioimmunoblastic (AILD, LgX)
T zone
Pleomorphic, small cell

**High grade T**
Pleomorphic, medium and large cell
Immunoblastic
Large cell anaplastic
Lymphoblastic

*Lancet* (1988) 292–293

For this reason many histopathologists continued to prefer one of the earlier schemes, and the Kiel classification came to be widely used, particularly in Europe. In hindsight it can be seen as the best of all the classification schemes proposed for non-Hodgkin's lymphoma. It introduced the idea of grading in terms of clinical aggressiveness. It also, when updated in 1988, listed neoplasms of B cell origin separately from T cell neoplasms.

The strength of the Kiel scheme lay in its correct identification, through careful microscopic examination, of many of the lymphoma categories which we recognize today. However, it went beyond basic observation and classification in its central concept that each stage of lymphoid cell maturation has a neoplastic equivalent. This led to the idea that certain lymphoma types *must* exist, since their normal counterparts had been identified.

# The Kiel Classification

| B Cell Lymphomas |
|---|

Lymphocytic

Centroblastic / centrocytic

Centrocytic

Centroblastic

Lymphoplasmacytoid

Immunoblastic

Lymphoblastic

**Bone Marrow**

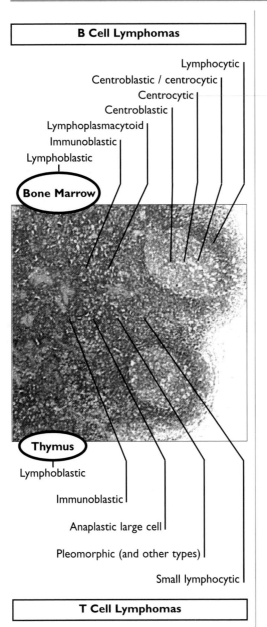

**Thymus**

Lymphoblastic

Immunoblastic

Anaplastic large cell

Pleomorphic (and other types)

Small lymphocytic

| T Cell Lymphomas |
|---|

Germinal Centers

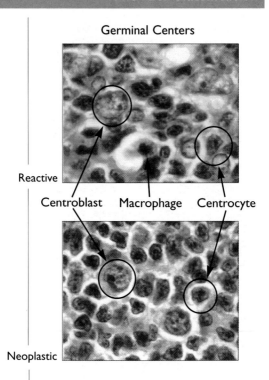

Reactive

Centroblast    Macrophage    Centrocyte

Neoplastic

The Kiel authors noted that follicular lymphoma contains a mixture of two neoplastic cell types which are essentially identical morphologically to cells in normal germinal centers. They suggested therefore that "centroblastic / centrocytic" lymphoma is the neoplastic counterpart of the germinal center, and evidence that has accumulated since that time fully confirms their view.

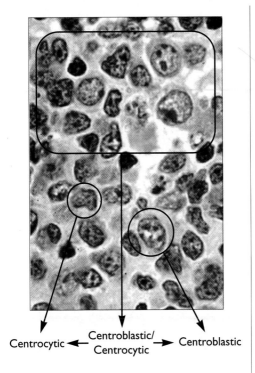

Centrocytic ←── Centroblastic/Centrocytic ──→ Centroblastic

They also proposed that "centroblastic/centrocytic" lymphoma lies within a spectrum, at one extreme of which is a lymphoma made up solely of centrocytes, and, at the other, a lymphoma comprising only centroblasts.

It is clear today however that the morphological similarity of "centrocytic lymphoma" to normal germinal cells is misleading. Similarly, there is no evidence that "centroblastic" lymphomas are related to the large transformed B cells of germinal centers, or indeed that they constitute a distinct lymphoma entity.

---

**A Revised European-American Classification of Lymphoid Neoplasms:**

**A Proposal from the International Lymphoma Study Group.**

Harris et al,
*Blood*, 84:1361–1392 (1994).

---

In 1994 the International Lymphoma Study Group published a consensus proposal for the classification of human lymphoid neoplasms, based on their shared experience in diagnostic hematopathology.

The Group is widely based, with approximately one third of its membership coming from the States and all but one of the remainder from different European countries. The classification contains no entities which have not been described extensively in the literature. It can be seen as an update of the Kiel scheme which removes some entities from which there is no good evidence and also includes extranodal lymphomas and Hodgkin's disease.

## International Lymphoma Study Group

Nancy Harris - Boston
Elaine Jaffe - Bethesda
Harald Stein - Berlin
Peter Banks - San Antonio
John Chan - Hong Kong
Michael Cleary - Stanford
Georges Delsol - Toulouse
Chris De Wolf-Peeters - Leuven
Brunangelo Falini - Perugia
Kevin Gatter - Oxford
Thomas Grogan - Tucson
Peter Isaacson - London
Daniel Knowles - Cornell
David Mason - Oxford
Konrad Müller-Hermelink - Würzburg
Stefano Pileri - Bologna
Miguel Piris - Toledo
Elizabeth Ralfkiaer - Copenhagen
Roger Warnke - Stanford

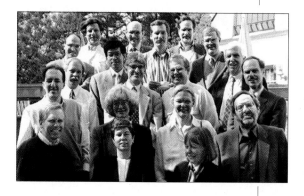

Ten of the non-Hodgkin's lymphomas in the REAL classification are of B lymphoid origin, and these are divided into those arising from immature cells, and those representing more mature B cells.

# B Cell Neoplasms

**Precursor B cell neoplasms**

Precursor B lymphoblastic
    leukemia / lymphoma

**Peripheral B cell neoplasms**

B cell chronic lymphocytic leukemia/
    prolymphocytic leukemia/
    small lymphocytic lymphoma

Immunocytoma / lymphoplasmacytic lymphoma

Mantle cell lymphoma

Follicle center lymphoma, follicular

Marginal zone B cell lymphoma

Hairy cell leukemia

Plasmacytoma / plasma cell myeloma

Diffuse large B cell lymphoma

Burkitt's lymphoma

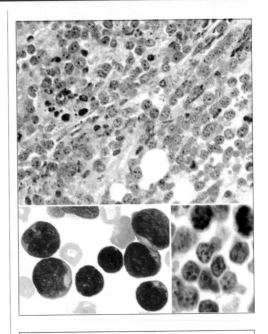

| Morphology | Lymphoblasts | |
|---|---|---|
| **Immunology** | TdT | + |
| | CD10 (CALLA) | + / - |
| | Cytoplasmic μ | - / + |
| | CD19, 79a | + |
| **Genetics** | No consistent abnormality | |
| **Clinical** | Children >> adults | |
| | Aggressive disease but | |
| | frequently curable | |

# B Lymphoblastic Leukemia / Lymphoma

Lymphoblastic neoplasms of B cell type usually present as a leukemia. They typically express markers, such as tèrminal transferase and CD10, found on early B cells. The CD79a antigen is of value, since it is often the only B cell marker expressed by these cells which is detectable in paraffin embedded tissue. Although bone marrow and blood involvement is very common, a few cases are localized as solid tumors, usually in lymph nodes. The disease, though aggressive, can be cured, particularly when it occurs in children.

Official name: "Precursor B lymphoblastic leukemia/ lymphoma"

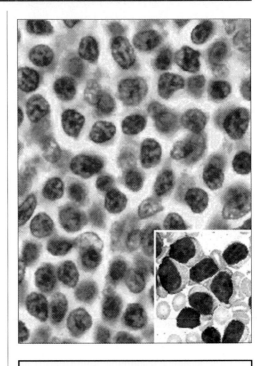

| Morphology | Predominantly small lymphocytes | |
|---|---|---|
| **Immunology** | Surface IgM | + (wk) |
| | CD5 | + |
| | CD10 | – |
| | CD19, 20, 79a | + |
| | CD22 | + / - |
| | CD23 | + |
| **Genetics** | Trisomy 12 or 13q abnormalities in some cases | |
| **Clinical** | Usually leukemic. Adults. Indolent course | |

# B Cell Small Lymphocytic Lymphoma

Neoplasms composed of small lymphocytes may also present as either lymphomas or leukemias. The leukemias comprise both chronic lymphocytic leukemia and the leukemia of larger cells which hematologists define as "prolymphocytic" leukemia.

Histologically, small lymphocytic neoplasms show a monotonous infiltration of small cells, but clusters of larger cells ("pseudofollicles or proliferation centers") are a common feature. Occasionally the neoplastic cells may differentiate to the plasma cell stage but this should not prompt a diagnosis of immuno-cytoma (see next page). Small lymphocytic neoplasms usually express CD5 and CD23, in addition to "pan-B cell" markers. They tend to follow an indolent course.

Includes chronic lymphocytic and pro-lymphocytic leukemia but the latter may be a clinically distinct entity.

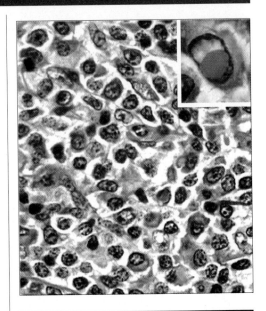

| Morphology | Plasmacytoid lymphocytes, plasma cells (+ / - Dutcher bodies), lymphocytes |
|---|---|
| Immunology | Surface IgM      + <br> Cytoplasmic Ig    + <br> CD5, 10         − <br> CD19, 20, 22, 79a   + |
| Genetics | No specific abnormalities |
| Clinical | Adults. Indolent course |

## Immunocytoma

The neoplastic cell in immunocytoma (also known as lymphoplasmacytic lymphoma) is a B lymphocyte, which shows a tendency to differentiate towards the plasma cell stage. IgM is detectable in the cells with plasmacytic features, within the cytoplasm or as intranuclear inclusions (Dutcher bodies). IgM may also appear in the serum as a paraprotein, and the disease then corresponds to Waldenström's macroglobulinemia. Strong cytoplasmic IgM positivity can help to distinguish the disease from small lymphocytic neoplasms, as does the absence of CD5.

Often associated with a serum IgM paraprotein

The disease is normally indolent but may transform to an aggressive large cell lymphoma. Other B cell neoplasms (e.g. small lymphocytic lymphoma and MALT lymphoma) may show plasmacytoid differentiation, and a diagnosis of immunocytoma should only be made in cases lacking features of these other lymphomas.

Mantle cell lymphoma is sometimes referred to as "intermediate lymphocytic lymphoma". It was first identified by the Kiel group as "centrocytic" lymphoma and their original description of its morphologic appearance cannot be bettered.

---

**Histologic appearance**

Small to medium sized cells, often with irregularly angular nuclei, and scant pale cytoplasm.

Occasionally the neoplastic cells are larger ("blastoid" variant).

The growth pattern is sometimes diffuse but more commonly a nodular or mantle zone pattern is seen.

A disordered array of dendritic reticulum cells is seen, contrasting with the prominent expanded nodular array seen in follicular lymphoma.

**Clinical features**

Excess of male patients. Median age 60. Frequent spread to blood and bone marrow. Median survival: less than 5 years.

---

Spread to the peripheral blood and to the bone marrow is commonly seen.

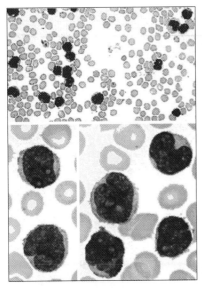

Blood

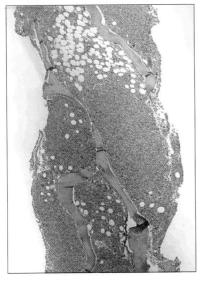

Bone marrow

Its pattern of antigenic expression is distinctive, as was first apparent more than ten years ago.

> "On detailed immunohistological analysis, it becomes apparent that there are many differences between centrocytic lymphoma and follicular CB-CC... Our immunological data support the view that centrocytic lymphoma is a separate entity, clearly distinguishable in most cases from other lymphoma categories."
>
> Stein H., Lennert K., Feller A.C. and Mason D.Y.
> *Advances in Cancer Research* (1984)
> 42: 67–147

CD5 is commonly present, but the disease differs from other CD5-positive B cell neoplasms (small lymphocytic lymphoma/leukemia) in lacking CD23. Cyclin D1 expression is common and can be diagnostically valuable.

| Phenotype | | |
|---|---|---|
| | Mantle cell lymphoma | Follicle center lymphoma | Small lymphocytic lymphoma/ leukemia |
| CD5 | Pos | Neg | Pos |
| CD10 | Neg | Pos | Neg |
| CD23 | Neg | Neg | Pos |
| Light chain | $\lambda > \kappa$ | $\kappa > \lambda$ | $\kappa > \lambda$ |
| Cyclin D1 | Pos | Neg | Neg |

The survival of cases of mantle cell lymphoma is unusual, in that it shows the steady fall characteristic of a relatively benign neoplasm (e.g. follicular lymphoma), reflecting a constant year-on-year mortality. However the slope is steep, and there is little indication of a plateau, as seen in large cell lymphomas. More aggressive therapy is usually of little benefit and long term survival is poor.

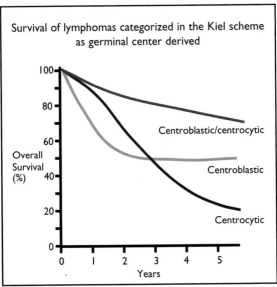

Based on data from The Non-Hodgkin's Lymphoma Classification Project
*Blood* (1997) 89: 3909–3918

Mantle cell lymphoma is associated with a characteristic cytogenetic anomaly, the (11;14) reciprocal chromosomal translocation. This anomaly is present in the majority of cases and causes over-expression of the BCL-1 or PRAD 1 gene, which encodes cyclin D1.

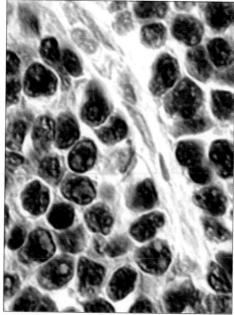

Cyclin D1 staining in lymphoma cells carrying the (11;14) translocation.

## Mantle Cell lymphoma

In the light of these clinical, immunological and genetic data, the disease was given the name "mantle cell lymphoma" by the International Lymphoma Study Group and it retains this name in the REAL scheme.

---

**Mantle cell lymphoma:**
**A proposal for unification of morphologic, immunologic and molecular data.**

Banks P., Chan J., Cleary M., Delsol G.,
De Wolf-Peeters C., Gatter K., Grogan T.,
Harris N., Isaacson P., Jaffe E., Mason D.,
Pileri S., Ralfkaier E., Stein H. and Warnke R.
(International Lymphoma Study Group).
*Amer. J. Surg. Pathol.* (1992) 16: 637–640

---

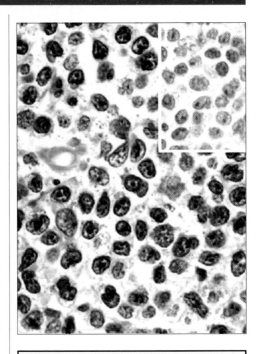

| Morphology | Small irregularly shaped centrocyte-like cells | |
|---|---|---|
| Immunology | Surface Ig (lλk) | + |
| | CD5 | + |
| | CD10 | - /+ |
| | CD19, 20, 22, 79a | + |
| | CD23 | − |
| | Cyclin D1 | + |
| Genetics | t(11;14). BCL-1 rearrangement | |
| Clinical | Adults. Moderately aggressive course (median survival 3–4 yrs) | |

## Mantle Cell Lymphoma

This change in nomenclature reflects the lack of evidence that the neoplastic cells derive from a germinal center cell (as the term "centrocytic" implied), and the realization that they have many of the features of mantle zone lymphocytes.

The disease usually presents with lymphadenopathy, but may be found at extranodal sites, notably the gastrointestinal tract (lymphomatous polyposis). The neoplastic cells are usually small to medium sized and may have irregular or "cleaved" nuclei, or a more "blastic" appearance. The growth pattern is often nodular and the neoplastic cells tend to "home" to the mantle zones of lymphoid follicles.

Equivalent to "centrocytic lymphoma" in Kiel scheme

# Follicle Center Cell Lymphoma

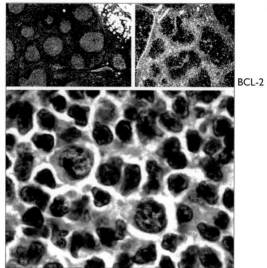

BCL-2

| | |
|---|---|
| **Morphology** | Mixture of germinal center blasts and cleaved cells (centroblasts and centrocytes). |
| **Immunology** | Surface Ig                 + <br> CD5                          – <br> CD10                     +/- <br> CD19, 20, 22, 79a   + <br> BCL-2                  + |
| **Genetics** | t(14;18) & *BCL-2* rearrangement in the majority of cases |
| **Clinical** | Adults. Indolent course (median survival 7–9 yrs) |

# Follicle Center Cell Lymphoma

Follicular lymphomas constitute, at least in the West, one of the most frequent non-Hodgkin's lymphomas, and it is clear that they are the neoplastic equivalent of normal germinal centers. This origin explains their title in the Kiel scheme of "centroblastic / centrocytic" lymphoma. They are usually easy to recognize because of their follicular growth pattern but they occasionally transform into diffuse tumors containing numerous large cells (centroblasts), and then fall into the group of "large B cell lymphoma".

The (14;18) chromosomal translocation, present in two-thirds to three-quarters of cases, juxtaposes the *BCL-2* gene to the Ig heavy chain gene, and this is accompanied by expression of BCL-2 protein. This is in contrast to normal germinal center B cells, which are BCL-2-negative. Follicular lymphomas which lack this translocation usually also express BCL-2 protein and show identical clinical behavior to translocation-positive cases. The disease is slowly progressive but essentially incurable.

Equivalent to "centroblastic/centrocytic" and "follicular centroblastic" lymphomas in the Kiel scheme

# Marginal Zone B Cell Lymphoma (MALT - type)

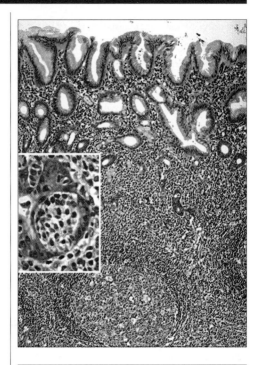

| Morphology | Small centrocyte-like cells, "monocytoid B cells", lymphocytes, plasma cells |
|---|---|
| Immunology | Surface Ig      + <br> CD5, 10      – <br> CD19, 20, 22, 79a   + <br> CD23      – |
| Genetics | t (11;18) in many cases. Trisomy 3 in some cases |
| Clinical | Indolent course, often localized. May transform to large cell lymphoma |

# Marginal Zone B Cell Lymphoma (MALT - type)

Marginal zone lymphomas are thought to represent the neoplastic equivalent of the marginal zone cells found in the spleen and lymph nodes, although, as in the case of mantle cell lymphoma, their origin is difficult to prove. The only marginal zone neoplasm unequivocally recognized in the REAL scheme is a small cell lymphoma. This arises in the gastrointestinal tract or other extra-nodal sites, usually glandular epithelial tissues, and is commonly referred to as "MALT lymphoma". These neoplasms derive from the B cells associated with epithelial tissues, and usually arise against a background of reactive lymphoid tissue, in which non-neoplastic germinal centers are prominent.

MALT lymphomas tend to remain localized, so that their prognosis is usually good, but they can transform to a large B cell lymphoma. When MALT lymphomas spread to mesenteric lymph nodes the possible appearance is identical to that of the rare "monocytoid B cell lymphoma". This latter disorder is a provisional entity in the REAL scheme, being classified as a sub-type of marginal zone B cell lymphoma. However some cases may represent nodal spread of an occult MALT lymphoma.

The REAL scheme includes nodal marginal zone lymphoma ("monocytoid B cell lymphoma") but as a provisional entity

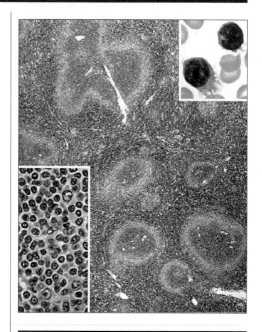

| Morphology | Small centrocyte-like cells, "monocytoid B cells", lymphocytes, plasma cells |
|---|---|
| Immunology | Surface Ig        +<br>CD5, 10       –<br>CD19, 20, 22, 79a  +<br>CD23           – |
| Genetics | No specific abnormalities |
| Clinical | Splenomegaly. ? Always leukemic |

# Splenic Marginal Zone B Cell Lymphoma

Splenic marginal zone lymphoma was included in the REAL scheme as another provisional subtype of marginal zone lymphoma. However, although there is now good evidence that it is a true clinicopathological entity, it is by no means certain that the neoplasm arises from marginal zone cells in the spleen. A major difference from marginal zone lymphoma of MALT type is the high incidence of bone marrow disease at presentation. This disease almost certainly corresponds to the rare form of chronic leukemia known by hematologists as "splenic lymphoma with villous lymphocytes".

Provisional entity in REAL scheme. Corresponds to "splenic lymphoma with villous lymphocytes"

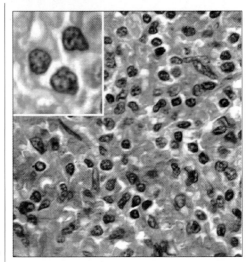

Spleen

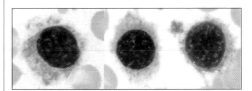

Blood

| | |
|---|---|
| **Morphology** | Small lymphoid cells with bean shaped nuclei and pale cytoplasm |
| **Immunology** | Surface Ig      + <br> CD5, 10, 23    − <br> CD11c, 25     + <br> CD19, 20, 22, 79a  + <br> CD103 (MLA)   + |
| **Genetics** | No specific abnormalities |
| **Clinical** | Adults, often with splenomegaly and pancytopenia. Indolent course |

## Hairy Cell Leukemia

Hairy cell leukemia is characterized by cells with fine villous surface projections and bean shaped nuclei, which are seen in the circulation, in the bone marrow and in the red pulp of the spleen. The latter sites of involvement account for pancytopenia and marked splenomegaly. Lymph node infiltration is rare.

The cells express, in addition to typical B cell antigens, the receptor for interleukin 2 (CD25) and the CD103 integrin (a cell adhesion molecule). In paraffin sections a distinctive pattern of markers can be detected, and these may be of diagnostic value, e.g. when the marrow shows a low level of infiltration. In addition to pan-B markers such as CD20 and CD79a, neoplastic cells often express CD68 (as cytoplasmic dots) and are labelled by antibody DBA.44. The disease tends to follow an indolent course.

# Plasmacytoma / Plasma Cell Myeloma

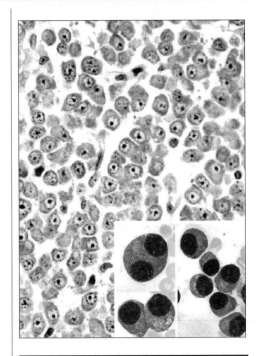

| Morphology | Plasma cells | |
|---|---|---|
| **Immunology** | Surface Ig | - |
| | Cytoplasmic Ig | + |
| | EMA | -/+ |
| | CD19, 20, 22 | - |
| | CD79a | +/- |
| **Genetics** | t(11;14) in a few cases | |
| **Clinical** | Adults. Lytic bone lesions, less commonly soft tissue tumor. Relapse after plateau phase | |

# Plasmacytoma / Plasma Cell Myeloma

Plasma cells are the cells characteristic of myeloma or plasmacytoma, the former term being used when the neoplasm is found in the bone marrow, causing skeletal destruction, and the latter for the rarer tumors which arise in soft tissue.

Usually associated with a serum paraprotein and / or urinary light chain excretion

B cell surface antigens are generally absent, in keeping with their loss by normal mature plasma cells, but cytoplasmic Ig (of a single light chain type) is present, accompanied in about 50% of cases by CD79a, one of the two chains of the molecule associated with Ig in B cells. The chromosome abnormality associated with mantle cell lymphoma, the (11;14) translocation, is found in some cases.

Patients with multiple myeloma usually respond initially to therapy, but almost all relapse after a period of remission.

**Centroblastic lymphoma:** Believed to derive from the germinal center, and to represent one end of the "centroblastic centrocytic spectrum."

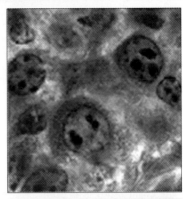

**Immunoblastic lymphoma:** Thought to belong to a B cell maturation pathway (found in extrafollicular areas of the lymph node), which leads to plasma cell production.

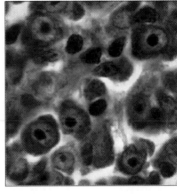

The Kiel scheme contains a third B cell neoplasm that was thought to be of germinal center origin, "centroblastic lymphoma". It was distinguished from the other category of diffuse high grade B cell neoplasm, "immunoblastic lymphoma", on the basis of a belief that the latter lymphoma arises from B cells which mature outside the B cell follicle. However, there is no convincing evidence for the validity of the distinction between "centroblastic" and "immunoblastic" lymphomas.

## Diffuse Large B Cell Lymphoma

It has been claimed that "immunoblastic" and "centroblastic" lymphomas show different survival curves, but this has not been confirmed in most studies. Furthermore there are no specific chromosome or genetic changes which can distinguish between these two diseases.

> "The difficulty in morphologically differentiating centroblastic lymphoma from immunoblastic lymphoma has caused a great deal of confusion, leading a number of lymphoma experts to suggest that the two categories should be included in a single group of 'large cell lymphoma'.
>
> "This immunohistological study only revealed minor differences between centroblastic lymphoma and immunoblastic lymphoma."
>
> Stein H., Lennert K., Feller A.C. and
> Mason D.Y. *Advances in Cancer Research* (1984) 42: 67–147

Equally importantly, pathologists have difficulty in reproducibly distinguishing between the proposed subtypes. Furthermore, as was first apparent more than 10 years ago, phenotypic studies do not provide evidence for such a distinction.

# Diffuse Large B Cell Lymphoma

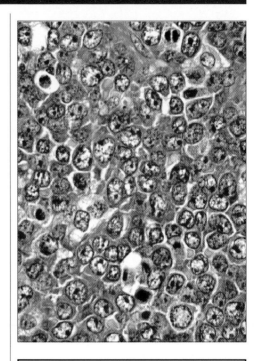

| Morphology | Monomorphous large cells with prominent nucleoli and basophilic cytoplasm |
|---|---|
| Immunology | Surface Ig        +/- <br> Cytoplasmic Ig    -/+ <br> CD5, CD10      -/+ <br> CD19, 20, 22, 79a   + |
| Genetics | t(14;18) in approx 30% <br> BCL-6 rearranged (40%) <br> and / or mutated (75%) |
| Clinical | Children or adults. Aggressive course, but may be curable |

## Diffuse Large B Cell Lymphoma

"Diffuse large B cell lymphoma" was therefore introduced in the REAL scheme to combine the "centroblastic" and "immunoblastic" categories.

It is one of the commonest categories of non-Hodgkin's lymphoma. Pan-B cell markers are expressed, and in a minority of cases the (14;18) chromosomal translocation is present, suggesting an origin from follicular lymphoma. The disease usually requires aggressive treatment, but may respond well, at least for a period.

The REAL scheme recognizes primary mediastinal (thymic) lymphoma as a rare subtype of large B cell lymphoma. The neoplastic cells often have characteristic pale cytoplasm and are thought to arise from intrathymic B cells. "Burkitt-like" lymphoma, however, probably represents a morphological appearance sometimes seen in diffuse large B cell lymphoma, and is probably not a distinct entity.

Combines "centroblastic" and "immuno-blastic" categories from Kiel scheme

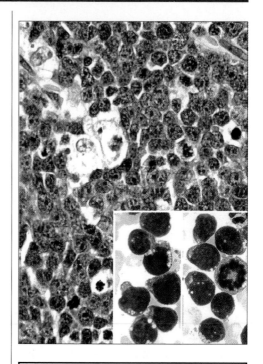

| Morphology | Medium sized cells, basophilic cytoplasm. "Starry sky" appearance. High mitotic rate | |
|---|---|---|
| Immunology | Surface IgM | + |
| | CD5, 23 | – |
| | CD10 | + |
| | CD19, 20, 22, 79a | + |
| | Ki67 | >85% of cells |
| Genetics | t(2;8), t(8;14) or t(8;22) Rearrangement of c-*MYC* | |
| Clinical | Children >> adults. Aggressive but curable in children | |

# Burkitt's Lymphoma

This tumor is typically made up of medium sized B cells with a high proliferation fraction, interspersed with macrophages containing cellular debris, giving the characteristic "starry sky" appearance. It may be difficult to distinguish with certainty from diffuse large cell lymphoma.

The immunophenotype is that of a peripheral B cell, although CD10 is also often present, which has prompted suggestions that it derives from germinal center cells.

In most "endemic" African cases Epstein–Barr viral DNA is found in the malignant cells. Histologically and phenotypically identical cases are also seen occasionally in the West. These may arise in patients with AIDS, and the EB virus is detectable in almost half of these cases. Non-African "sporadic" cases also arise in the absence of immune impairment, and EB virus is detectable in less than a quarter of these cases.

Almost all cases, from whatever country, show a chromosomal translocation involving the *MYC* gene on chromosome 8 and the gene for Ig heavy chain or, less commonly, one of the two Ig light chain genes. The disease may respond to aggressive therapy.

"Burkitt-like" lymphoma is a provisional entity in the REAL scheme, but many pathologists currently interpret this as a morphological appearance seen in some diffuse larger B cell lymphomas, and not a distinct entity

The other major category of lymphoid neoplasia in the REAL scheme (apart from Hodgkin's disease) comprises those arising from T cell or natural killer cells. As in the case of the B cell disorders, they are subdivided in the REAL scheme into lymphoblastic neoplasms, which arise from immature cells of thymic origin, and those which arise from differentiated peripheral T cells.

# T Cell and Natural Killer Cell Neoplasms

**Precursor T cell neoplasm**

Precursor T lymphoblastic
leukemia / lymphoma

**Peripheral T cell and NK cell
neoplasms**

T cell chronic lymphocytic leukemia/
prolymphocytic leukemia

Large granular lymphocyte leukemia (LGL)

Mycosis fungoides / Sézary syndrome

Peripheral T cell lymphomas, unspecified

Angioimmunoblastic T cell lymphoma (AILD)

Angiocentric lymphoma

Intestinal T cell lymphoma

Adult T cell lymphoma / leukemia (ATL/L)

Anaplastic large cell lymphoma (ALCL)

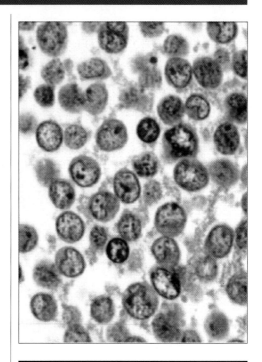

| Morphology | Lymphoblasts, identical cytologically to B lymphoblasts |
|---|---|
| Immunology | TdT       + <br> CD1a    +/- <br> CD3     +/- <br> CD7     + <br> CD4 ± 8  + |
| Genetics | *SCL / TAL*-1 rearrangement in approx 25% |
| Clinical | Frequently involves mediastinum. Adolescents and young adults. Highly aggressive but potentially curable |

# T Lymphoblastic Leukemia / Lymphoma

The morphology of lymphoblastic neoplasms of precursor T cell origin is usually indistinguishable from that of B cell lymphoblastic neoplasms. They typically present as acute leukemias but occasionally give rise to tumors in the lymph node or thymus. T cell antigens are present although CD3 is usually, because of the immaturity of the cells, only found in the cytoplasm. The disease is potentially curable with aggressive therapy.

REAL name: "Precursor T lymphoblastic lymphoma/ leukemia"

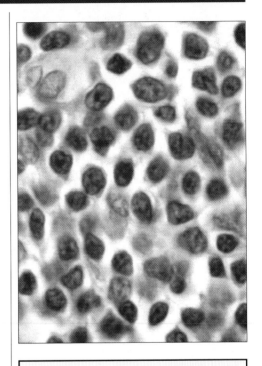

| Morphology | Small lymphoid cells, with some nuclear irregularity |
|---|---|
| Immunology | CD2, 3, 5, 7     +<br>CD4                +<br>CD8                -/+ |
| Genetics | Inv 14(q11;32) in 75%<br>Trisomy 8q |
| Clinical | Adults. Often leukemic. More aggressive than B cell chronic lymphocytic leukemia |

# T Cell Chronic Lymphocytic Leukemia

T cell lymphomas of small lymphocytes resemble small lymphocytic B cell neoplasms in that they often involve the peripheral blood, and their morphology is similar. Their nucleoli may be more prominent and the cytoplasm more abundant, so that some cases would be classified hematologically as "prolymphocytes" and this category includes cases that hematologists would categorize as T cell prolymphocytic leukemia. However, debate about whether there is a true distinction between prolymphocytic and chronic lymphocytic leukemia of T cell origin is largely academic, given their rarity and the generally poor prognosis.

Unlike small lymphocytic B cell lymphoma, pseudofollicles containing larger cells are not seen. These lymphomas express pan-T cell antigens and also CD7, and are commonly CD4-positive. The disease tends to follow a more aggressive course than small lymphocytic B cell tumors.

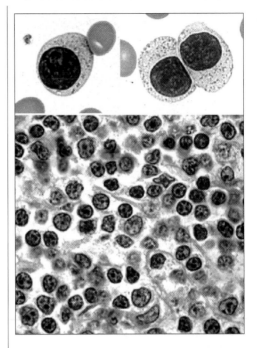

| Morphology | Small to medium lymphoid cells with eccentric round or oval nuclei. Azurophilic cytoplasmic granules |
|---|---|
| Immunology | CD2 + |
| | CD3, 8 +/- |
| | CD16 + |
| | CD56, 57 -/+ |
| Genetics | No specific abnormalities |
| Clinical | Adults, usually leukemic. Neutropenia ± anemia. Indolent course |

# Large Granular Lymphocyte Leukemia

Neoplasms arising from "large granular lymphocytes" can be subdivided, on the basis of phenotype, into those which arise from T cells and those which probably derive from natural killer cells.

*T cell type:* This disease is usually indolent, and patients may be asymptomatic. Other cases present with recurrent infection due to neutropenia, and 25% of patients have clinical features of rheumatoid arthritis. The prognosis is usually good.

*NK cell type:* Patients are younger (median age 40 years) and symptoms are more acute (e.g. fever, B symptoms). Massive hepatosplenomegaly, involvement of the GI tract and coagulopathy may occur. In contrast, arthritis and symptomatic neutropenia are rare. The disease tends to follow an aggressive course.

The borderline is not always clear between Asian cases of NK cell leukemia and angiocentric (nasal) lymphomas.

Two types —

T cell:
  CD3+
  CD56-
  CD57+/-

NK cell:
  CD3-
  CD56+/-
  CD57+/-

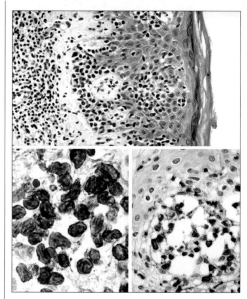

| Morphology | Small to medium sized cells with cerebriform nuclei epidermal infiltration |
|---|---|
| Immunology | CD2, 3, 4, 5  + <br> CD7, 8, 25  − |
| Genetics | No specific abnormalities |
| Clinical | Adults. Principally localized to skin but may involve blood and lymph nodes |

# Mycosis Fungoides / Sézary Syndrome

Mycosis fungoides is a T cell lymphoma seen most commonly in the skin, but which is referred to as Sézary syndrome when the characteristic cells are also found in the circulation. The neoplastic cells accumulate in the epidermis, where they may form localized pockets referred to as "Pautrier's micro-abscesses", and have a typical convoluted cerebriform nuclear morphology. As the disease progresses it can spread to lymph nodes, where the interfollicular zones are infiltrated.

Phenotype may change as disease progresses

The cells express pan-T cell antigens and are almost always of CD4 "helper" subtype. In many cases a number of the neoplastic T cells also express CD30 which can be a useful feature to distinguish it from dermatitis.

The disease follows a variable course but may become widespread and has a tendency to transform to a large cell tumor.

Although a number of well defined categories of T cell neoplasia have come to be recognized over the years (e.g. mycosis fungoides/ Sézary syndrome), many T cell tumors have none of the features of these subtypes. They were often referred to as "pleomorphic" or "polymorphic" T cell neoplasms, reflecting their wide variation in cell morphology.

---

### Kiel Classification of T Cell Lymphomas

**A. Prethymic and thymic leukemia / lymphoma**
Lymphoblastic

**B. Peripheral T cell lymphoma / leukemia**
*Low grade*
Chronic lymphocytic and prolymphocytic leukemia
Small cerebriform cell (mycosis fungoides/ Sézary syndrome)
Lymphoepithelioid (Lennert's lymphoma)
Angioimmunoblastic (AILD, LgX)
T zone
Pleomorphic, small cell (HTLV-1 ±)
*High grade*
Pleomorphic, medium and large cell (HTLV-1 ±)
Immunoblastic (HTLV-1 ±)
Large cell anaplastic

Suchi T, Lennert K. *et al. J. Clin. Pathol.* 1987; 40: 995.

---

A revision of the Kiel scheme in 1987 defined two subtypes of pleomorphic T cell neoplasms, one (of low grade) made up of small cells and the other (of high grade) containing medium and large lymphoma cells. A category of immunoblastic T cell neoplasia was also proposed.

## T Cell Lymphomas in the Kiel Scheme

Many pathologists found it difficult to apply this new aspect of the Kiel classification scheme to diagnostic samples. This became clear in a study by a group of Danish hematopathologists who were unable in practice to use the Kiel criteria in a reproducible fashion for diagnosing T cell neoplasms.

---

**Peripheral T Cell Lymphomas:**
**an evaluation of reproducibility of the updated Kiel Classification**

100 peripheral T cell lymphomas studied.

"A low inter-observer reproducibility was found."

"Our study confirms the problems of defining reproducible morphological criteria for classifying lymphomas."

"The updated Kiel classification for T cell lymphomas fails to satisfy the requirement for adequate reproducibility."

Hastrup N., Hamilton-Dutoit S., Ralfkiaer E. and Pallesen G. *Histopathology* (1991) 18: 99–105.

---

For this reason the REAL scheme created a single category of "peripheral T cell lymphoma". The word "unspecified" was added to indicate that this category may comprise several entities.

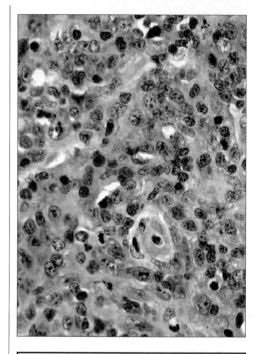

| | |
|---|---|
| **Morphology** | Atypical lymphocytes of varying sizes. Variable reactive background elements, e.g. macrophages, vessels, etc. |
| **Immunology** | CD3          +/- <br> Variable expression of other T cell markers. |
| **Genetics** | No specific abnormalities |
| **Clinical** | Adults. Aggressive course but potentially curable |

## Peripheral T Cell Lymphoma, Unspecified

These neoplasms typically contain a mixture of small and large neoplastic cells, often with irregular nuclei. There may be a marked infiltration of non-neoplastic cells, including macrophages and eosinophils. In some cases, clusters of epithelioid histiocytes, characteristic of so-called "Lennert's" or lymphoepithelioid T cell lymphoma, are seen.

A variety of patterns of T cell antigen expression is found, CD4 being more frequent than CD8. Peripheral T cell lymphomas are for some reason seen with greater frequency in the Far East than in Europe and the United States, where they account for less than 20% of non-Hodgkin's lymphomas. The prognosis is very variable.

"Unspecified" reflects suspicion that subtypes (currently unidentifiable) exist

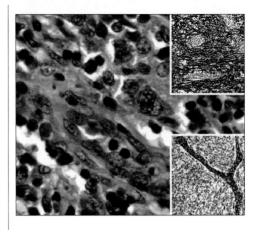

| Morphology | Architecture effaced, arborizing high endothelial venules, no secondary follicles. Mixed infiltrate of lymphocytes, blasts and atypical clear cells |
|---|---|
| Immunology | T cell phenotype. Large follicular dendritic cell clusters around proliferating venules |
| Genetics | No specific abnormalities |
| Clinical | Systemic disease with lymphadenopathy, fever, weight loss, and skin rash. Polyclonal hypergamma-globulinemia. Aggressive course |

# Angioimmunoblastic T Cell Lymphoma

Angioimmunoblastic T cell lymphoma was initially thought of as an abnormal immune reaction, but is now considered as a category of peripheral T cell lymphoma in which the neoplastic cells are mixed with and obscured by a complex histological picture including proliferating vessels, epithelioid histiocytes, plasma cells, eosinophils, and hyperplastic clusters of follicular dendritic cells. The neoplastic cells are of variable morphology and include atypical "clear" cells with indented nuclei and abundant pale cytoplasm. The cells carry T cell markers and are usually CD4-positive.

Patients often have systemic symptoms such as weight loss, fever, skin rash and a polyclonal hypergammaglobulinemia. The disease is moderately aggressive and a high grade lymphoma (usually of T but occasionally of B cell type) may emerge.

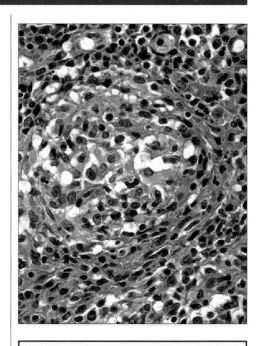

| Morphology | Polymorphic lymphocytes, infiltrating vessel walls |
|---|---|
| Immunology | CD2, 56 + <br> CD3 -/+ <br> CD5, 7 +/- <br> CD4 or 8 +/- |
| Genetics | No specific abnormalities |
| Clinical | Children and adults. Commoner in Asia than US / Europe. Extranodal sites involved, e.g. nose, palate, skin. Variable course |

# Angiocentric Lymphoma

A feature of this lymphoma which is also referred to as "nasal" or "nasal-type" lymphoma, is a tendency to invade the walls of blood vessels, accompanied in many cases by blockage of vessels by lymphoma cells, often associated with ischemic necrosis of normal and neoplastic tissue. The cell morphology is very variable, and admixed inflammatory cells may cause difficulty in diagnosing early cases.

Should be distinguished from lymphomatoid granulomatosis

EBV is almost always present in the neoplastic cells. The neoplastic cells are probably of natural killer cell rather than T cell origin: surface CD3 is absent in many cases (although cytoplasmic CD3 epsilon chain is present) and CD56 is often expressed.

The disease is rare in the United States and Europe, but is much commoner in Asia and often involves the nose, palate and skin but other soft tissues may also be involved. The distinction from Asian neoplasms of large granular lymphocytes is not always clear. The clinical course ranges from indolent to aggressive.

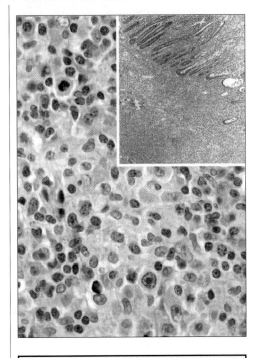

| | |
|---|---|
| **Morphology** | Neoplastic cells range from small lymphocytes to large bizarre cells |
| **Immunology** | CD3, 7       + <br> CD8         +/- <br> CD103 (MLA)   + |
| **Genetics** | No specific abnormalities |
| **Clinical** | Adults. Aggressive course, often with intestinal perforation |

## Intestinal T Cell Lymphoma

Small intestinal lymphomas have long been recognized as a complication of celiac disease. They were first thought to be a heterogeneous group of tumors but later studies suggested a histiocytic origin. In the early 1980s it became clear that they were T cell lymphomas of widely varying morphology.

This neoplasm is often associated with small bowel ulceration. The typical histological features of celiac disease, though often present, may be absent due to the phenomenon of "latency" recently recognized in celiac patients. In keeping with this, some patients have a history of documented celiac disease while others present with the lymphoma.

The neoplastic cells express pan T cell markers and, in most cases, the CD103 integrin molecule found on normal intestinal T lymphocytes. The clinical outlook is poor since the neoplasm is frequently multifocal.

May be associated with celiac disease

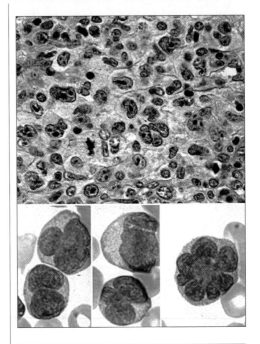

| | |
|---|---|
| **Morphology** | Pleomorphic infiltrate of small and large lymphoid cells |
| **Immunology** | CD2, 3, 4, 5, 25    +<br>CD7           – |
| **Genetics** | Integrated HTLV-1 genome present |
| **Clinical** | Adults. Commonest in Japan and Caribbean. Hypercalcemia, leukemia, bone lysis. Commonly aggressive; rarely indolent |

# Adult T Cell Lymphoma / Leukemia

In the 1970s, an unusual T cell neoplasm was reported in South Western Japan which was subsequently shown to be confined to patients infected with the HTLV-1 retrovirus. Identical cases were then found in other areas of HTLV-1 infection, notably the Caribbean.

The lymph node is diffusely replaced by neoplastic T cells, which vary widely in cell size and regularity, and neoplastic cells may also be seen in the peripheral blood. Patients often have aggressive disease, associated with lytic bone lesions, and hypercalcemia, but the course is very variable, and indolent or smoldering cases are seen.

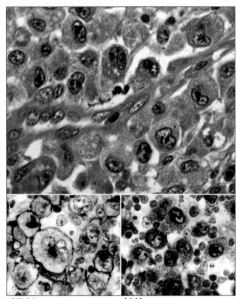

CD30                    ALK

| Morphology | Bizarre large cells, sometimes R-S like or multi-nucleate. Abundant cytoplasm. Cohesive cells, intrasinus spread |
|---|---|
| Immunology | T or null phenotype<br>CD30       +<br>EMA       +/-<br>ALK       +/- |
| Genetics | t(2;5), causing fusion of *ALK* and *NPM* genes, in majority of cases |
| Clinical | Systemic form aggressive but potentially curable. Rare primary cutaneous disease, mainly in adults, is more indolent but incurable |

# Anaplastic Large Cell Lymphoma

Anaplastic large cell lymphoma was first recognized as a neoplasm which was positive for the Ki-1 or CD30 antigen, an activation-associated antigen also found on Reed-Sternberg cells. The neoplastic cells tend to be larger than in any other type of lymphoma, and cases may be misdiagnosed as malignant histiocytosis or even anaplastic carcinoma. Distinction from Hodgkin's disease may also on occasion be difficult.

Typically the tumor grows in a cohesive pattern, tending to invade lymphoid sinuses. When cell lineage markers are present they indicate a T cell origin. A (2;5) translocation, causing fusion of the nucleophosmin (*NPM*) gene with a gene encoding the ALK receptor kinase may be present, and recent data suggest that this abnormality (detectable by immuno-staining for ALK protein) defines a distinct entity with a benign course.

The majority of cases (particularly those with the (2;5) translocation) are children or young adults. The clinical pattern is variable, some cases showing widespread involvement of lymph nodes and other sites, and other cases being confined to skin. The latter form of the disease is indolent but difficult to cure, whereas the systemic type may respond to aggressive treatment.

Sometimes referred to as "Ki-1 lymphoma"

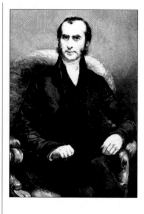

Thomas Hodgkin
(1798-1866)

Thomas Hodgkin described seven cases of lymphadenopathy whilst curator of the museum at Guy's Hospital in the 1830s. Examination of material from the four cases preserved at the museum has shown that two were definitely examples of Hodgkin's disease, one was probably a non-Hodgkin's lymphoma, and one was an inflammatory lesion, possibly tuberculosis.

Failing to get a consultant (staff) appointment at Guy's, Hodgkin turned to philanthropic activities which included founding the "Aborigines' Protection Society". He died in Jaffa of dysentery whilst visiting the Holy Land with his friend Sir Moses Montefiore.

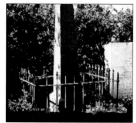

Hodgkin's grave
at Jaffa

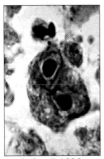
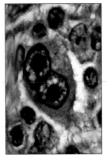

R-S cell 1830s        R-S cell 1990s

Sections of tissue from Hodgkin's original cases, preserved in alcohol for many years, show typical Reed-Sternberg cells. The remarkable cytological presentation of this material is complemented by the preservation of the Reed-Sternberg associated marker CD15.

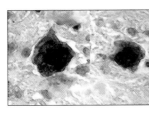

Original Hodgkin's case

CD15 staining

The Rye classification in the 1960s postulated four subtypes of Hodgkin's disease, and these have been incorporated virtually unchanged into the REAL scheme. The majority of cases, referred to as "classical Hodgkin's disease", fall into three categories (although the REAL scheme also identifies a provisional "lymphocyte-rich" category). These classical subtypes share features which distinguish them from lymphocyte predominance Hodgkin's disease.

**RYE - 1965**

    Nodular sclerosing
    Mixed cellularity
    Lymphocyte depletion
    Lymphocyte predominance

**REAL - 1994**

"Classical" types
    Nodular sclerosing
    Mixed cellularity
    Lymphocyte depletion
    Lymphocyte rich *

Lymphocyte predominance

             *Provisional

In classical Hodgkin's disease, scattered binucleate or multi-nucleate Reed-Sternberg cells and mononuclear Hodgkin's cells are associated with a reactive cellular infiltrate of lymphoid cells, eosinophils and other inflammatory cells.

The nodular sclerosing subtype is characterized by prominent fibrotic bands running through the diseased tissue, a thickened lymph node capsule and "lacunar" cells, a morphologic variant of the Reed-Sternberg cell created when the cell cytoplasm retracts within the surrounding fibrotic environment.

These features are absent in mixed cellularity Hodgkin's disease, in which the heterogeneous cellular infiltrate is the cardinal feature. When this infiltrate is sparse and Reed-Sternberg cells numerous and often bizarre, the disease falls into the lymphocyte depletion category, while the reverse pattern is seen in the provisional lymphocyte-rich category. The lymphocyte depletion subtype is rare and may be difficult to distinguish from anaplastic large cell lymphoma.

### Nodular Sclerosing

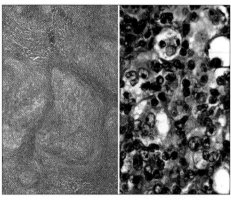

Low power         Lacunar cells

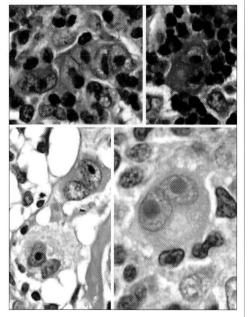

Reed-Sternberg cells

## Mixed cellularity

In mixed cellularity Hodgkin's disease the node contains a mixed infiltrate of abnormal and reactive cells. The infiltrate usually has a paracortical localization, as seen when remnants of crushed follicles are demonstrated by immunostaining for B cell antigens. When this pattern is marked, a diagnosis is sometimes made of "interfollicular" Hodgkin's disease. Apoptotic or "mummified" neoplastic cells are commonly found.

Low power H & E

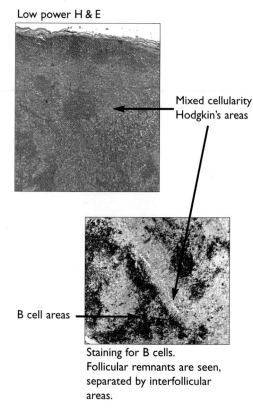

Mixed cellularity Hodgkin's areas

B cell areas

Staining for B cells.
Follicular remnants are seen, separated by interfollicular areas.

# Hodgkin's Disease: "Classical" Subtypes

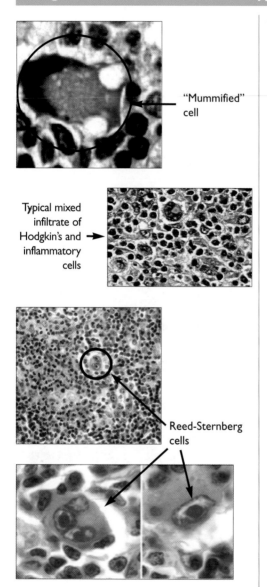

"Mummified" cell

Typical mixed infiltrate of Hodgkin's and inflammatory cells

Reed-Sternberg cells

## Lymphocyte predominance

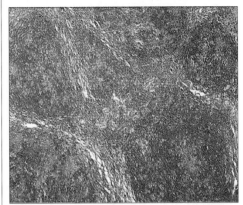

Low power

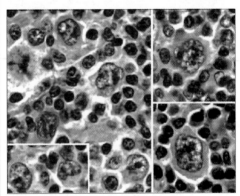

High power

In lymphocyte predominance Hodgkin's disease, as in the classical subtypes, scattered neoplastic cells are seen against the background of an abnormal cellular infiltrate. However, most of the neoplastic cells, known as "L & H" (lymphocytic and histiocytic) or "popcorn" cells, lie within large nodular areas made up of small lymphoid cells.

Immunostaining shows that the nodules contain extensive meshworks of follicular dendritic cells, and that the lymphoid cells are almost all polyclonal small B lymphocytes, expressing both IgM and IgD.

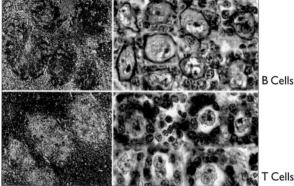

B Cells

T Cells

T cells are present in the nodules in much smaller numbers and many are found around the L & H cells.

This pattern clearly distinguishes lymphocyte predominance disease from other Hodgkin's subtypes, in which the background infiltrate is rich in T lymphocytes.

The phenotype of L & H cells is also different from that of classical Reed-Sternberg cells. They express, among other B cell markers, J chain, a protein which is found in Ig-secreting B cells but not in Reed-Sternberg cells. In contrast, although B cell antigens can be found on Reed-Sternberg cells in some cases of classical Hodgkin's disease, they are usually only found on a minority of the neoplastic cells.

## Cell Phenotype in Hodgkin's Disease

|  | Classical R-S cells | L & H cells |
|---|---|---|
| CD3 / TCRβ | Occasionally positive | Negative |
| CD15 | Usually positive | Usually negative |
| CD20 | Occasionally positive | Usually positive |
| Other B markers | Rarely positive | Frequently positive |
| CD30 (Ki-1) | Positive | Sometimes positive |
| CD45 (LCA) | Usually negative | Often positive |
| CDw75 (LN1) | Usually negative | Usually positive |
| EMA | Usually negative | Often positive |
| Ig | Polytypic or negative | Negative or monotypic |
| J chain | Negative | Positive |
| EBV genome | Frequently positive | Infrequently positive |

Lymphocyte predominance Hodgkin's disease is distinctive not only at the cellular level but also in its clinical manifestations. For example, it shows a striking male predominance and its pattern of spread differs from that of other Hodgkin's subtypes. It tends to be an indolent, slowly progressive disorder, although occasional cases transform after a period into large cell lymphoma, usually of B cell type.

The REAL scheme recognizes a total of more than 20 different lymphoid neoplasms, but may be simplified by listing separately those found mainly in lymph nodes and those seen at extranodal sites, and also by categorizing them according to cell morphology, rather than by cell lineage.

| Lymphoid neoplasms in lymph node biopsies | |
| --- | --- |
| **Neoplasm** | **Origin of neoplastic cell** |
| **Non-Hodgkin's** | |
| Small lymphocytic lymphoma / leukemia | B cell |
| Immunocytoma | B cell |
| Mantle cell lymphoma | B cell |
| Follicle center lymphoma | B cell |
| Burkitt's lymphoma | B cell |
| Diffuse large B cell lymphoma | B cell |
| Lymphoblastic lymphoma / leukemia | B cell |
| Peripheral T cell lymphoma | T cell |
| Adult T cell leukemia / lymphoma | T cell |
| Angioimmunoblastic T cell lymphoma (AILD) | T cell |
| Anaplastic large cell lymphoma | T cell or null |
| **Hodgkin's** | |
| Nodular sclerosing, mixed cellularity and lymphocyte depletion | ? B cell |
| Lymphocyte predominance | B cell |

This gives a total of eleven categories of non-Hodgkin's lymphoma in lymph node samples, excluding provisional categories, plus Hodgkin's disease.

## Extranodal and Nodal Lymphomas

Six entities are seen principally at extranodal sites. "Splenic marginal zone B cell lymphoma" and "mediastinal B cell lymphoma" may be added since, despite their provisional status, they seem to be clearly defined entities.

| Neoplasm | Type | Common sites |
|----------|------|--------------|
| Hairy cell leukemia | B cell | Spleen and bone marrow |
| Plasmacytoma / myeloma | B cell | Bone marrow |
| MALT lymphoma | B cell | Gut and other epithelial sites |
| Intestinal T cell lymphoma | T cell | Small intestine |
| Angiocentric lymphoma | T cell | Nose, palate and elsewhere |
| Mycosis fungoides/ Sézary syndrome | T cell | Skin |

Non-Hodgkin's lymphomas differ greatly in incidence and in the US and Europe large B cell lymphomas and follicular lymphoma account together for two-thirds of cases.

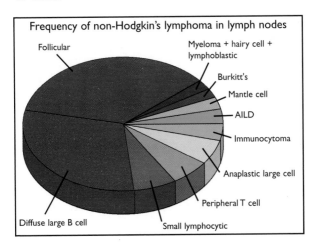

Frequency of non-Hodgkin's lymphoma in lymph nodes

Follicular

Myeloma + hairy cell + lymphoblastic

Burkitt's

Mantle cell

AILD

Immunocytoma

Anaplastic large cell

Peripheral T cell

Small lymphocytic

Diffuse large B cell

The publication in 1994 of the REAL scheme prompted a major multicenter evaluation of its practical utility and clinical implications. A total of approximately 1400 non-Hodgkin's lymphomas were submitted from nine institutions in eight countries.

| Centre | Number of cases |
|---|---|
| Omaha | 200 |
| Vancouver | 202 |
| Cape Town | 196 |
| London | 120 |
| Locarno | 80 |
| Lyon | 195 |
| Hong Kong | 200 |
| Würzburg / Göttingen | 210 |

All cases were reviewed by five expert hematopathologists, only one of whom was a member of the International Lymphoma Study Group responsible for the REAL scheme.

# NHL Classification Project

## Visiting hematopathologists

J. Diebold (Paris)
K.A. MacLennan (Leeds)
H. K. Müller-Hermelink (Würzburg)
B. N. Nathawani (Los Angeles)
D. Weisenberger (Omaha)

## Consultant hematopathologist

N. L. Harris (Boston)

The study aimed to determine

-   the ability of hematopathologists to apply the ILSG classification

-   the role of immunophenotyping and clinical data in diagnosis

-   the clinical importance of immunophenotyping

-   the reproducibility of diagnosis

-   clinical correlations and whether certain entities can be grouped for prognostic or therapeutic purposes.

The Non-Hodgkin's Lymphoma Classification Project
*Blood* (1997) **89**: 3909–3918

Each hematopathologist recorded an initial diagnosis, based solely on histology (first diagnosis), and could then revise this opinion on the basis of clinical and immunophenotypic data (final diagnosis).

| Consensus diagnosis | First diagnosis (%) | Final diagnosis (%) |
|---|---|---|
| Follicular | 93 | 94 |
| Marginal zone B-cell, MALT | 84 | 86 |
| Small lymphocytic (CLL) | 84 | 87 |
| Immunocytoma | 53 | 56 |
| High grade B-cell, Burkitt-like | 47 | 53 |
| Mediastinal large B-cell | 51 | 85 |
| Marginal zone B-cell, nodal | 55 | 63 |
| Mantle cell | 77 | 87 |
| Diffuse large B-cell | 73 | 87 |
| Precursor T-lymphoblastic | 52 | 89 |
| Anaplastic large T / null-cell | 46 | 85 |
| Peripheral T-cell, all types | 41 | 86 |

The Non-Hodgkin's Lymphoma Classification Project.
*Blood* (1997) 89: 3909–3918

For most lymphoma categories the final diagnosis agreed well with the group's consensus diagnosis. There were three exceptions — immunocytoma, nodal marginal zone lymphoma and Burkitt-like large cell lymphoma — suggesting that better criteria may be required, or even that these may not represent true disease entities.

# NHL Classification Project

For some categories (e.g. follicular lymphoma) the correct diagnosis was usually made on the basis of conventional histologic examination alone, but other lymphoma types (e.g. anaplastic large cell lymphoma) required immunophenotypic and / or clinical data, as shown by the differing figures for initial and final diagnosis.

> "For 94% of the cases re-reviewed... the expert pathologists made a diagnosis consistent with either their original diagnosis or the consensus diagnosis. In only 6% of the cases... the pathologist's re-review diagnosis would likely have led to a different approach to therapy than the original diagnosis."
>
> The Non-Hodgkin's Lymphoma Classification Project. *Blood* (1997) 89: 3909–3918

Twenty per cent of cases were re-reviewed to assess whether the expert hematopathologists could repeat their original diagnosis, and this showed a reassuringly high level of consistency.

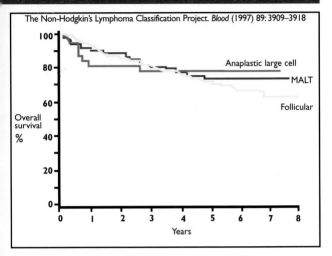

The Non-Hodgkin's Lymphoma Classification Project. *Blood* (1997) 89: 3909–3918

After confirmation of the validity of the REAL scheme the clinical behavior of each case was reviewed. The best prognosis group comprised three entities with an overall 5-year survival of greater than 70%.

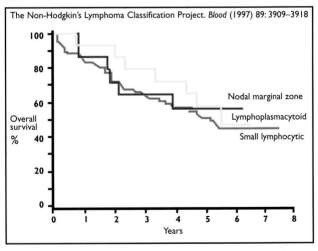

The Non-Hodgkin's Lymphoma Classification Project. *Blood* (1997) 89: 3909–3918

A second category comprised lymphomas with a 5-year survival of 50 to 70%.

## Lymphoma Prognosis

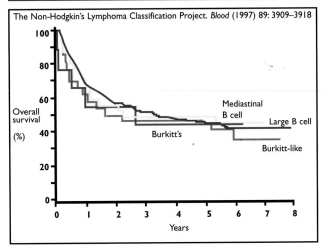

The Non-Hodgkin's Lymphoma Classification Project. *Blood* (1997) 89: 3909–3918

Lymphomas with a 5-year survival of 30–50% included the controversial "Burkitt-like" lymphoma, whose survival curve is essentially identical to that of large B cell lymphoma.

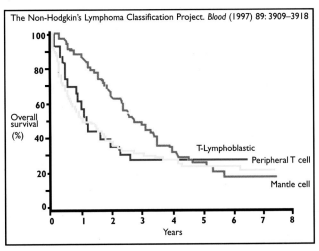

The Non-Hodgkin's Lymphoma Classification Project. *Blood* (1997) 89: 3909–3918

The group of lymphomas with the poorest prognosis included mantle cell lymphomas. Initially the prognosis is better than for other poor risk lymphomas, but after five years is worse.

This study also emphasized the importance of both histopathologic and clinical features when assessing a new case of lymphoma. In follicular lymphoma, for example, the International Prognostic Index, based on factors such as serum LDH and disease bulk, defines clinical subgroups with strikingly different prognoses.

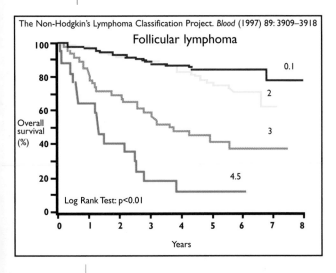

The Non-Hodgkin's Lymphoma Classification Project. *Blood* (1997) 89: 3909–3918

Follicular lymphoma

Log Rank Test: p<0.01

The Non-Hodgkin's Lymphoma Classification project therefore validated the REAL classification as a scheme which can be reproducibly applied by hematopathologists. It also documented the clinical features of each category and underlined the relevance of clinical assessment.

# The WHO Classification

A comprehensive classification of all neoplasms of hemopoietic and lymphoid tissue is currently being prepared under the auspices of the World Health Organisation. Extensive discussions, involving 10 subcommittees and input from a Clinical Advisory Committee, have already taken place concerning non-Hodgkin's lymphoma.

It appears that no new entities which are not covered by the REAL scheme are envisaged, and that the list of lymphoid neoplasms in the WHO scheme is likely to be essentially identical to the REAL scheme. However, the WHO scheme will probably include a few rare disorders which were provisional categories in the REAL scheme (e.g. hepatosplenic $\gamma\delta$ and panniculitic lymphomas among the T cell tumors, and nodal marginal zone lymphomas among the B cell neoplasms). The WHO scheme may also subdivide some entities in the REAL scheme (e.g. distinguishing prolymphocytic B cell leukemia from small lymphocytic B cell neoplasms, and listing plasmacytoma separately from plasma cell myeloma and Sézary syndrome from mycosis fungoides).

Immunohistological staining of paraffin sections may be needed to assign non-Hodgkin's lymphomas to B or T cell lineage or when morphological features are difficult to interpret e.g. when the sample is small or badly processed. On occasion, it may not even be certain that the neoplasm is of lymphoid origin.

*B cell neoplasms:* The markers of choice are CD20 and CD79a. These pan-B cell markers give very similar reactions, although CD79a appears earlier in B cell maturation, and can be used to detect precursor B cell lymphoblastic neoplasms, and is found on some plasma cell neoplasms when CD20 is lost. Other B cell markers, such as CDw75, are less specific and their reactions should be interpreted with care.

*T cell neoplasms:* CD3 is the most widely used marker since it is never found on B cells. It is occasionally lost by neoplastic T cells, so that alternative markers such as CD43 or CD45RO, although not specific for T cells, may be of supplementary value. However, these antigens are also found in some B cell lymphomas and can be expressed by macrophages and myeloid cells.

| Marker | Specificity |
|---|---|
| **B cells** | |
| CD20 | Virtually B cell specific but negative on precursor B cells |
| CD45RA | Antigen also found on some T cells |
| CDw75 | Also on other epithelial cells |
| CD79a | Essentially B cell specific |
| Immunoglobulin | B cell specific but may be obscured by background Ig |
| **T cells** | |
| CD3 and TCR | T cell specific but lost by some neoplastic cells |
| CD8 | Specific for cytotoxic/suppressor cells |
| CD43 | Antigen also present on some B cells, myeloid cells and macrophages |
| CD45R0 | Also present on myeloid cells, macrophages and some B cells |
| TIA-1, granzyme B, perforin | Markers of cytotoxic T cells |

*Other markers:* A variety of other molecules (see next page) may be of use for the diagnosis of lymphoproliferative disorders.

**Myeloid**

| | |
|---|---|
| CD15 | Also found on Reed-Sternberg cells, epithelium, etc. |
| CD66 | Also present on epithelial cells |
| CD68 | Pan-macrophage |
| Elastase | Specific for neutrophil lineage |
| Lysozyme | Neutrophil / macrophage marker, also found in secretory cells |

**Oncogene products**

| | |
|---|---|
| BCL-1 | Confirmatory marker of mantle cell lymphoma |
| BCL-2 | Follicular lymphoma and many other neoplasms |
| BCL-6 | Marker of diffuse large B cell, follicular and Burkitt's lymphoma, and of LPHD |
| ALK | Marker of t(2;5)-positive lymphomas |

**Miscellaneous**

| | |
|---|---|
| TdT | Marker of lymphoblasts |
| CD21 | Follicular dendritic cell marker |
| CD30 | Marker of Reed-Sternberg cells and ALCL |
| CD31 | Megakaryocyte / platelet and endothelial marker |
| CD45 (LCA) | Essential for carcinoma/ lymphoma distinction |
| CD61 (GPIIIA) | Marker of platelets and megakaryocytes |
| CD74 / MHC Class II | Marker of B cells, some macrophages, and IRC |
| DBA.44 | Marker of hairy cell leukemia |

---

### CONCLUSION

**There is now broad agreement among hematopathologists over the lympho-proliferative disorders which they recognize.**

These entities correspond in many respects to the Kiel classification, with three major exceptions:

a) "Large cell B cell lymphoma" replaces "centroblastic" and "immunoblastic".

b) A major category of unspecified peripheral T cell lymphomas is created by uniting several subgroups.

c) Extranodal lymphomas and Hodgkin's disease are included.

---

The REAL classification represents a new initiative which should resolve many of the disagreements which have complicated the nomenclature and identification of human lymphoid neoplasms in the past. Unlike other schemes, it does not categorize these tumors clinically as high or low grade, because it is now recognized that each entity has its own characteristic pattern of behavior.

---

The REAL classification represents what hematopathologists **do**, not what they **should** do.

---

# Index

## H

Hairy cell leukemia 36–7
Higby, D.J. 5
Hodgkin, Thomas 70
Hodgkin's cells 74
Hodgkin's disease 70–81, 83
  classical 74–6
  interfollicular 76
  in lymph node biopsies 82
  lymphocyte depletion 74
  lymphocyte predomi-
    nance 78–80
  lymphocyte-rich 74, 79
  mixed cellularity 74, 76–7
  nodular sclerosing 74, 75
HTLV-I 66, 67

## I

Immunoblastic lymphoma
  40–3
immunoblastic T cell
  neoplasms 56
immunocytoma 20–1
immunoglobulin (Ig) 81, 93
  heavy chain 31
  light chain 39, 45
immunoglobulin M (IgM) 21
interleukin 2 receptor
  (CD25) 37
intermediate lymphocytic
  lymphoma 22
International Lymphoma
  Study Group 12–13
intestinal T cell lymphoma
  64–5

## J

J chain 80, 81

## K

Kay, Humphrey E.M. 3
Kiel classification 2, 7–11, 95
  T cell neoplasms 9, 56–7
Ki-I (CD30) 55, 69, 81, 94

## L

L & H (lymphocytic and
  histiocytic) cells 78–81
lacunar cells 74
large B cell lymphoma 25, 31
  diffuse 40–3
large granular lymphocytic
  leukemia 52–3
Lennert's T cell lymphoma 59
Lukes / Collins classification 2
lymph node biopsies 82
lymphoepithelioid T cell
  lymphoma 59
lymphomatous polyposis 29
lymphoplasmacytic lymphoma
  20–1
lysozyme 94

## M

MALT lymphoma 32–3
mantle cell lymphoma 22–9,
  89
marginal zone B cell
  lymphoma
  extranodal 32–3
  nodal 33
  splenic 34–5
mediastinal lymphoma,
  primary 43
monocytoid B cell lymphoma
  32, 33
mummified cells 76, 77
MYC gene 45
mycosis fungoides 54–5
myeloid antigens 94
myeloma, plasma cell 38–9

## N

Nasal lymphoma 63
natural killer (NK) cell
  neoplasms 46–47, 53, 63
non-Hodgkin's lymphoma
  classification schemes
  6–7, 14–15, 46–7

# Index

# Captain Cook

## THE GREAT OCEAN EXPLORER

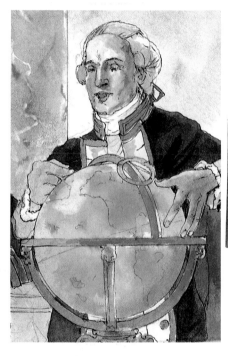

## HAYDN MIDDLETON

### Illustrated by Alan Marks

OXFORD UNIVERSITY PRESS

James Cook was born in 1728, in the village of Marton in the north of England. His family did farm work, and they lived in a small cottage with earth walls on the edge of the Yorkshire moors.

As James grew up, he helped on the farm. But he also learned to read and write, and became very good at arithmetic. When he had any free time, he went down to the coast to watch the ships passing by. They were carrying coal down to London, where King George II had his court.

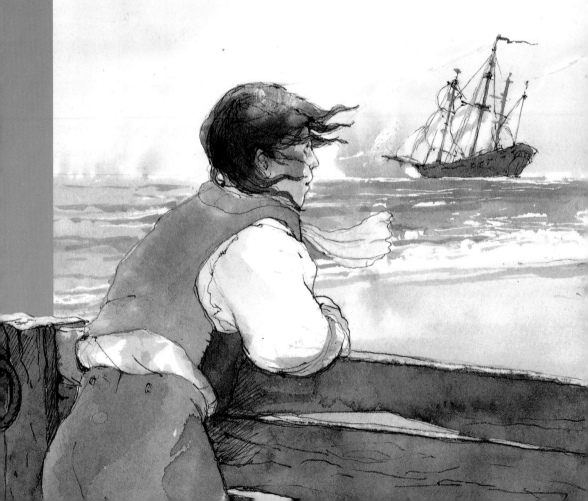

James loved to gaze out to sea. His secret dream was to be a sailor. He longed to visit London, and cities in foreign countries as well. Perhaps he might even travel on a ship to lands that nobody yet knew about.

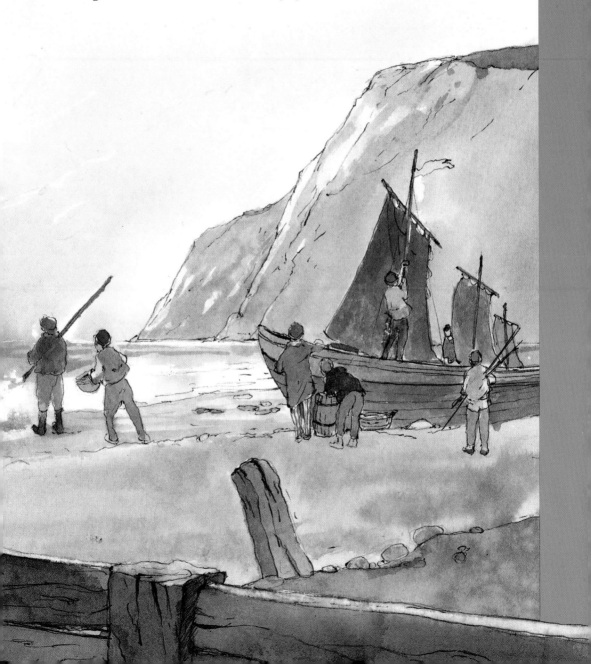

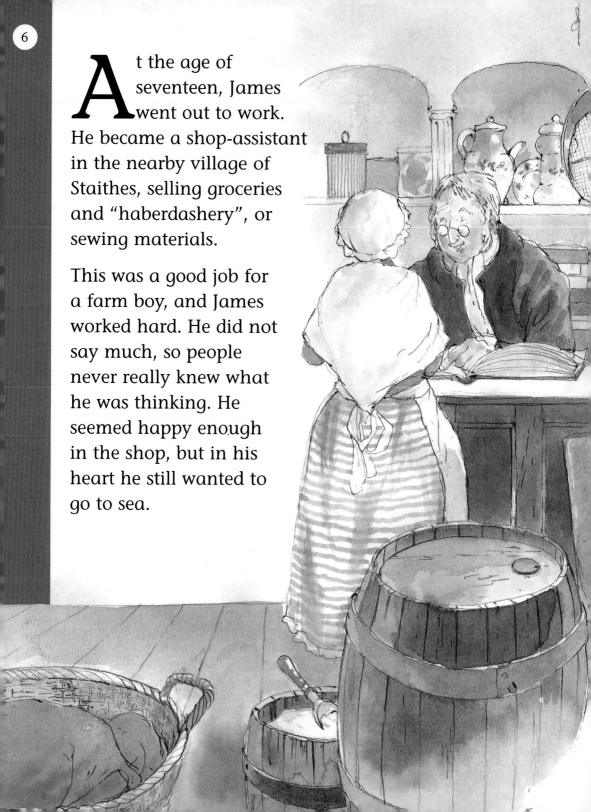

At the age of seventeen, James went out to work. He became a shop-assistant in the nearby village of Staithes, selling groceries and "haberdashery", or sewing materials.

This was a good job for a farm boy, and James worked hard. He did not say much, so people never really knew what he was thinking. He seemed happy enough in the shop, but in his heart he still wanted to go to sea.

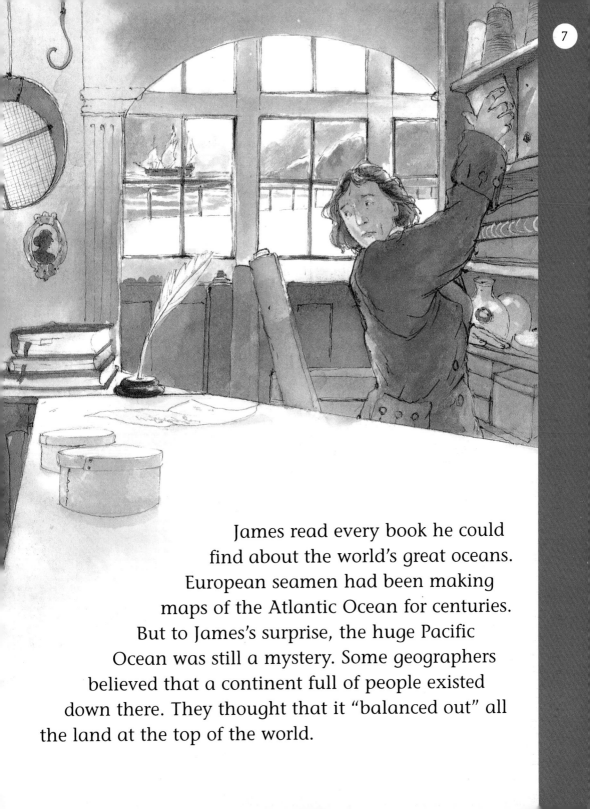

James read every book he could
find about the world's great oceans.
European seamen had been making
maps of the Atlantic Ocean for centuries.
But to James's surprise, the huge Pacific
Ocean was still a mystery. Some geographers
believed that a continent full of people existed
down there. They thought that it "balanced out" all
the land at the top of the world.

When James was eighteen, he decided to follow his dream. He gave up his job at the shop and became an apprentice to John Walker, a coal-ship owner at the local port of Whitby. At last he was going to sea – as a Ship's Boy.

James was big and strong for his age. He also had to be brave, because life on the coal ships could be tough and dangerous. But James loved every minute of it, and between voyages he read book after book about "navigation", the science of keeping ships on course.

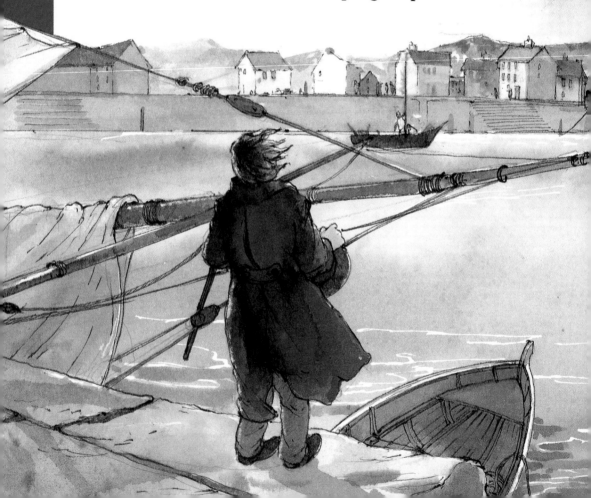

John Walker was pleased with James – he was always so calm and reliable. In 1755 he asked James to take command of a coalship. But James had other plans. Britain was about to fight a war against France. James joined the Navy, and three years later he was crossing the Atlantic Ocean to Canada as Ship's Master, in charge of navigation on *HMS Pembroke*.

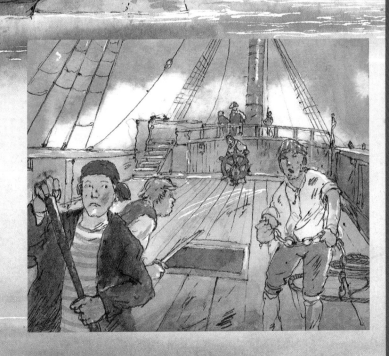

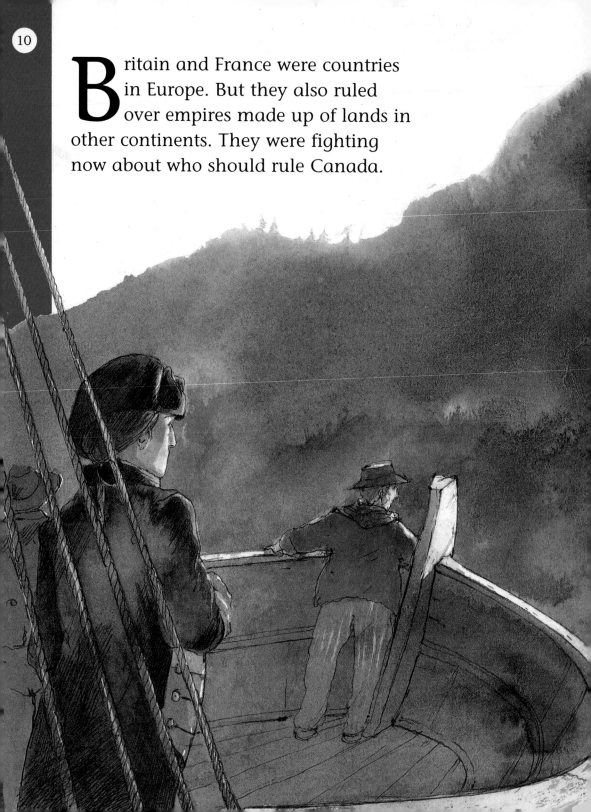

Britain and France were countries in Europe. But they also ruled over empires made up of lands in other continents. They were fighting now about who should rule Canada.

One dark night in 1759, James had a vital job to do. Ships carrying British soldiers were sailing up Canada's St Lawrence River. They planned to make a surprise attack on the great French fortress of Quebec. James, the expert navigator, had to map out a safe path for the warships to follow.

This was not easy. The river was wide, fast-flowing and full of rocks. But James calmly guided all the soldiers as far as Quebec. There they rushed ashore, captured the fortress, then went on to seize the whole of Canada. James's map of the St Lawrence River was so good, people were still using it a hundred years later.

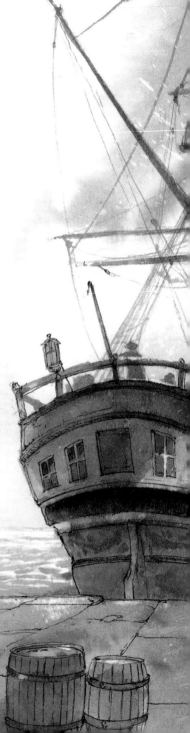

After the war James returned to London. He was now 34 years old. Most men of that age were already married. James had been so busy since joining the Navy, there had been no time to find a wife.

In 1762 James married a woman called Elizabeth Batts, the daughter of a shopkeeper. They set up home together and soon started a family. But James was hardly ever at home. He spent the next five summers far across the Atlantic Ocean, making detailed maps of Canada's coastlines for the Navy.

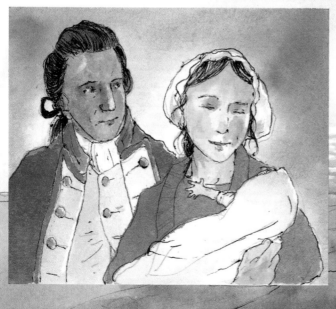

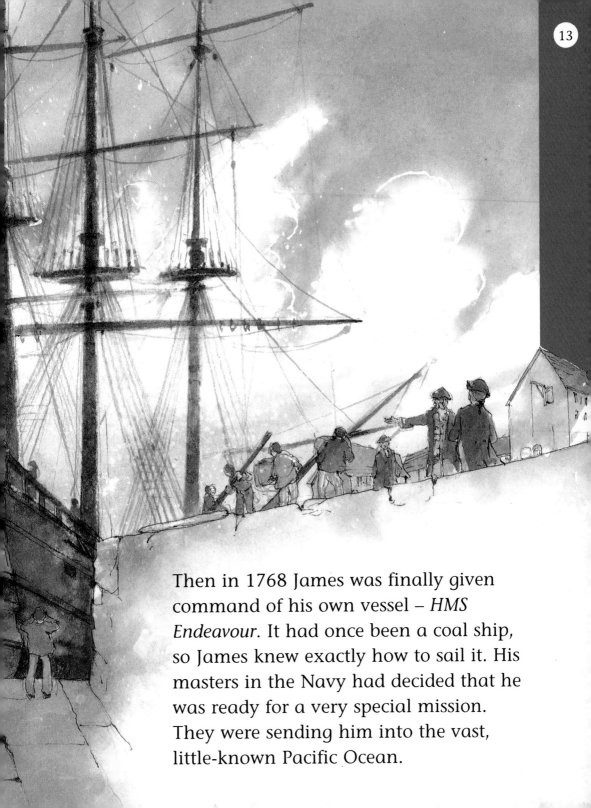

Then in 1768 James was finally given command of his own vessel – *HMS Endeavour*. It had once been a coal ship, so James knew exactly how to sail it. His masters in the Navy had decided that he was ready for a very special mission. They were sending him into the vast, little-known Pacific Ocean.

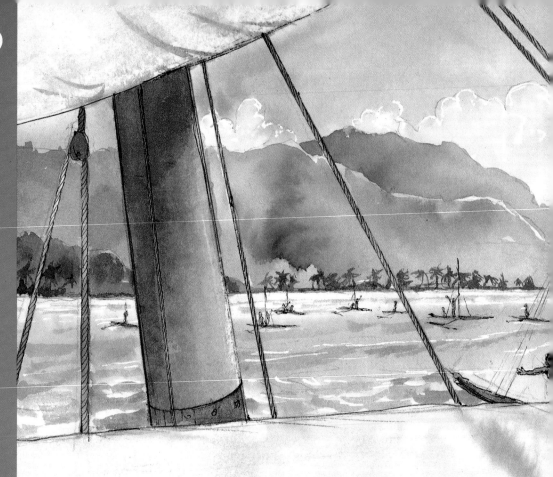

The *Endeavour* set sail from Plymouth on 26 August 1768. The ship was only 32 metres long, but it had to carry ninety-four men. Some of them were famous scientists. They hoped to sail to the Pacific island of Tahiti. There they would watch the "Transit of Venus" – the movement of the planet Venus across the Sun. That was the official purpose of the expedition.

But James also had some secret orders. He was to search for the Great Southern Continent, which no European had ever found.

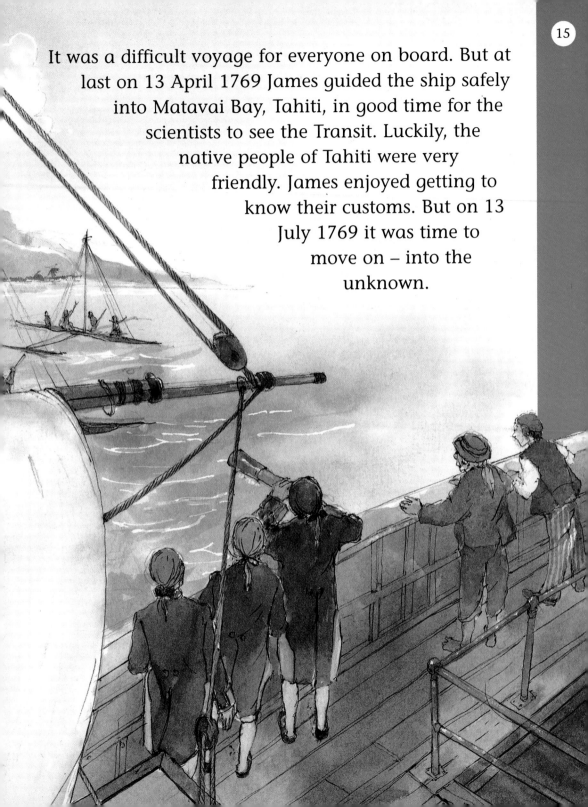

It was a difficult voyage for everyone on board. But at last on 13 April 1769 James guided the ship safely into Matavai Bay, Tahiti, in good time for the scientists to see the Transit. Luckily, the native people of Tahiti were very friendly. James enjoyed getting to know their customs. But on 13 July 1769 it was time to move on – into the unknown.

The *Endeavour* sailed west then south. After three months, a large mass of land loomed ahead. It was New Zealand, which had first been seen by Dutch sailors in 1642. Was this a part of a Great Southern Continent? Before James could find out, the local people – the Maoris – made a fierce attack on the *Endeavour*.

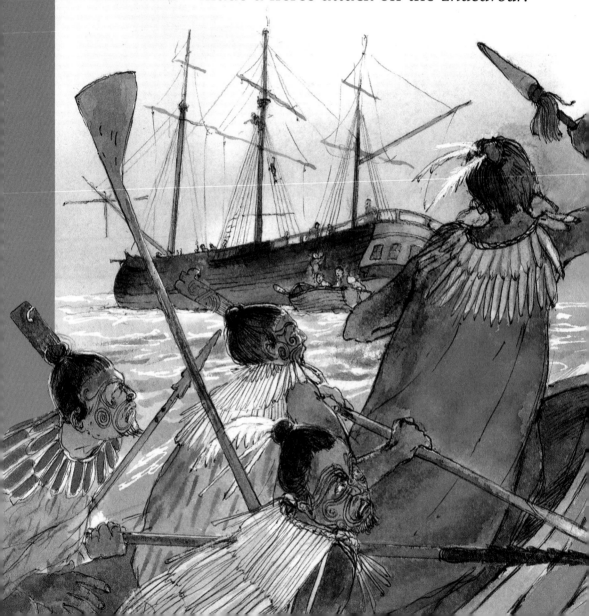

*Endeavour's* crew managed to beat off the Maori war canoes, but they had to stay on constant alert for more attacks. James was unafraid. He took the ship carefully along the coasts, making a map as he went. New Zealand turned out to be made up of two islands.

Heading west again, James found another shore and began to map it. One place was so full of new plants he called it Botany Bay (botany is the study of plants). His men also spotted some strange hopping animals – kangaroos. James called this wonderful land New South Wales, because it reminded him of Wales in Britain. Later, it would be known as Australia.

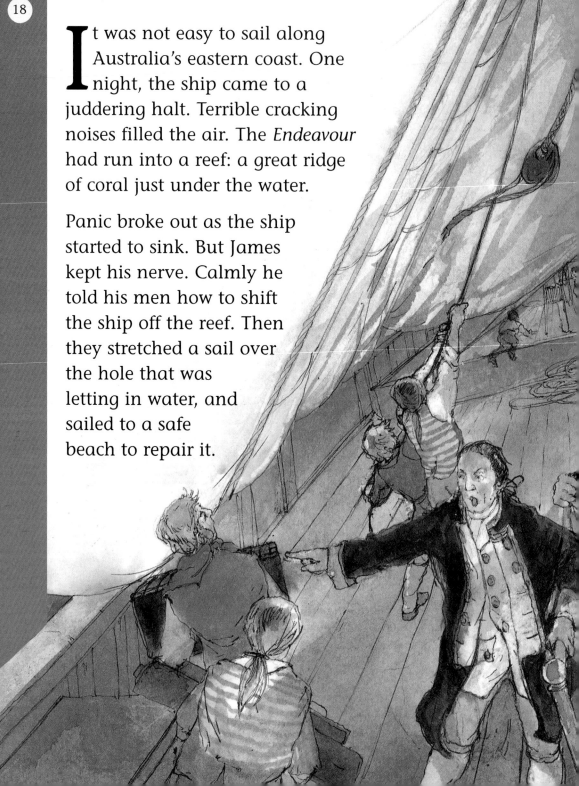

It was not easy to sail along Australia's eastern coast. One night, the ship came to a juddering halt. Terrible cracking noises filled the air. The *Endeavour* had run into a reef: a great ridge of coral just under the water.

Panic broke out as the ship started to sink. But James kept his nerve. Calmly he told his men how to shift the ship off the reef. Then they stretched a sail over the hole that was letting in water, and sailed to a safe beach to repair it.

When the hole was mended, the *Endeavour* sailed back home to England. The expedition had lasted for three years. Usually on long voyages, many men died of a disease called scurvy, caused by their poor diet. But James had provided healthy food, so his crew was not badly affected.

The voyage had been a huge success. James's report of it made him very famous. Soon New Zealand and Australia were added to the British Empire. But still no one knew for sure if a Great Southern Continent existed.

AUSTRALIA

'Endeavour' ran aground here

NEW ZEALAND

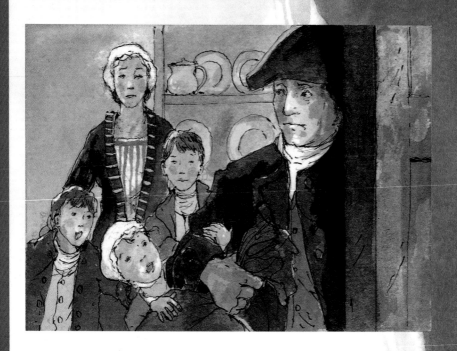

James spent only a year at home with his family. He was promoted again, to Commander, and in July 1772 he set out on a second voyage. Again his mission was to find out if there really was a Great Southern Continent. This time there were two ships. James commanded the *Resolution*. Tobias Furneaux was in charge of the *Adventure*.

The two ships called at Capetown in southern Africa, then headed off in search of the southern continent. But the further south they sailed, the worse the weather became. The crews had never known such cold – even the special warm clothing that James had brought for them did not keep out the chill.

The ships zigzagged past huge icebergs until at last a great sea of ice blocked their path. James now knew the truth. If a southern continent existed, it could only be in these frozen wastes known as the "Antarctic" – and no people could possibly live there.

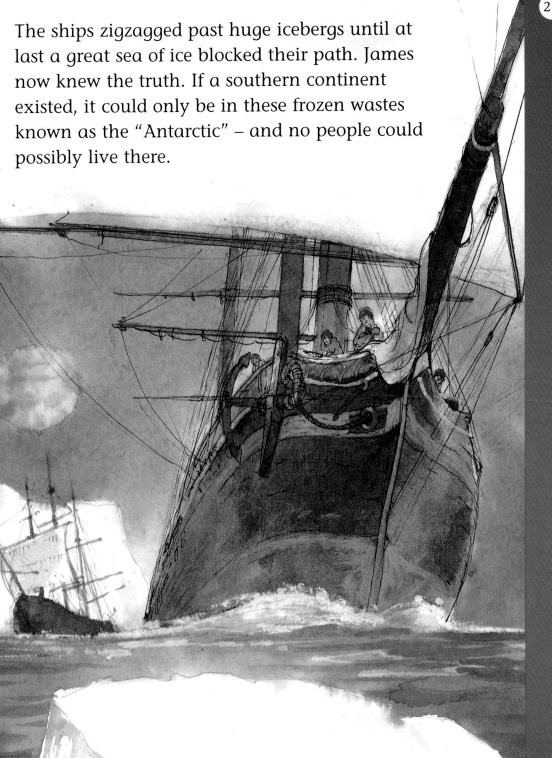

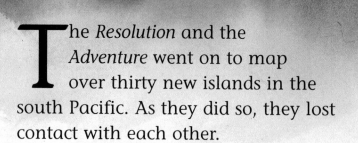

The *Resolution* and the *Adventure* went on to map over thirty new islands in the south Pacific. As they did so, they lost contact with each other.

James and his crew were glad to be back in the warm ocean after almost freezing in their search for the southern continent. One of the most mysterious places they visited was Easter Island. On the grassy slopes of this lonely island, massive stone heads had been carved. Some of them were over nine metres tall. Nobody knew what they were for.

When the *Resolution* reached Tahiti, the island's big war fleet put on a show. The Tahitians, like most of the islanders in the Pacific, were friendly to the British sailors. But the Melanesians at Erromanga threw stones and fired arrows. And in New Zealand, James found that something much worse had happened to some of the *Adventure*'s crew.

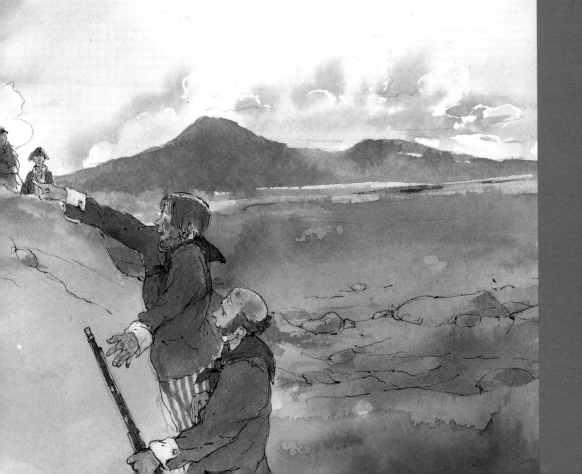

The *Resolution* called in at New Zealand on its way home. There James was horrified to learn that Maori cannibals had attacked, killed and eaten ten crewmen from the *Adventure*. The *Adventure* had then returned to England, becoming the first ship ever to sail around the world from west to east.

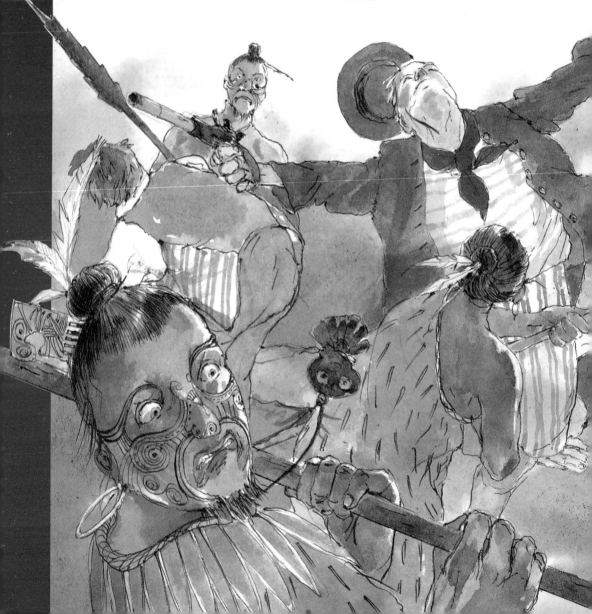

James and his men followed in the *Resolution*. Throughout this voyage they were able to stay on course more accurately than ever before, because James had brought along a brand new piece of equipment to help him navigate.

This was a "chronometer", a sea clock invented by John Harrison. The Navy had asked James to test it, and he found that it was very accurate. He called it his "Watch Machine, our never failing guide". It guided James and the *Resolution* back to England in July 1775. There he was met with a hero's welcome.

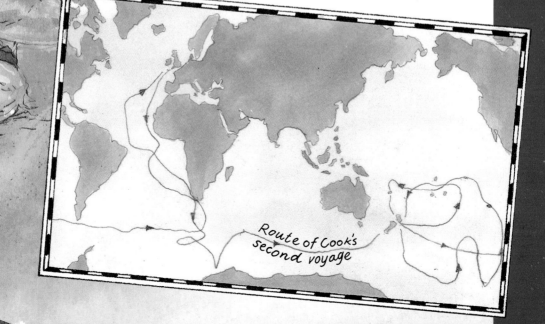

Route of Cook's second voyage

James had been ill for a while on the second voyage. He was now 46, which was quite old in those days. And he had spent seven of the last eight years at sea. He believed that his days of adventure were over, and planned to spend the rest of his life quietly with his wife and three children.

He was well rewarded for his explorations. He was promoted to "Captain" Cook. The Royal Society – an important club for scientists – made him a member. He was even invited to court, where he was presented to King George III.

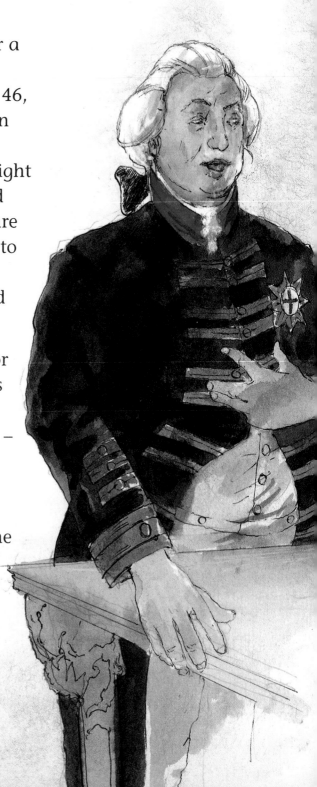

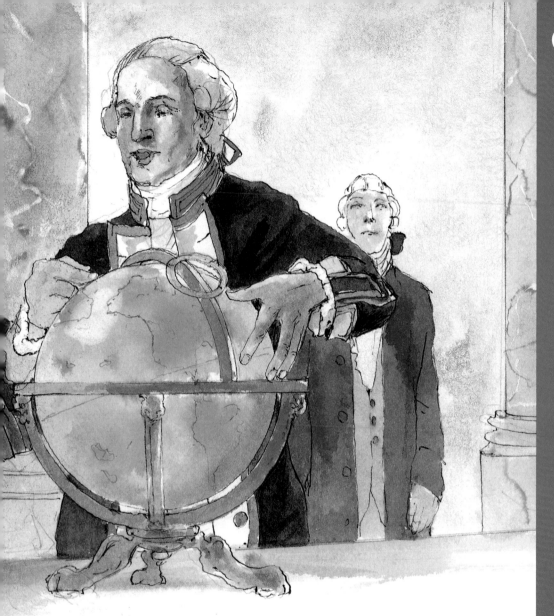

Then in 1776, the Navy organized a new expedition. Its aim was to see if there was a "North-West Passage", or route from the Pacific to the Atlantic across the top of America. The Earl of Sandwich asked James who he thought should be put in command. James smiled and said he would do the job himself.

In July 1776, the *Resolution* set sail from Plymouth. James called his ship "A Noah's Ark". On board were all sorts of farm animals, to be used for breeding in faraway lands. A second ship, the *Discovery*, was commanded by Charles Clerke.

They went first to New Zealand. James left some rabbits and goats with the Maoris. Then he moved on to Tahiti, and afterwards the Hawaiian Islands, which he had not visited before. The people there greeted him warmly.

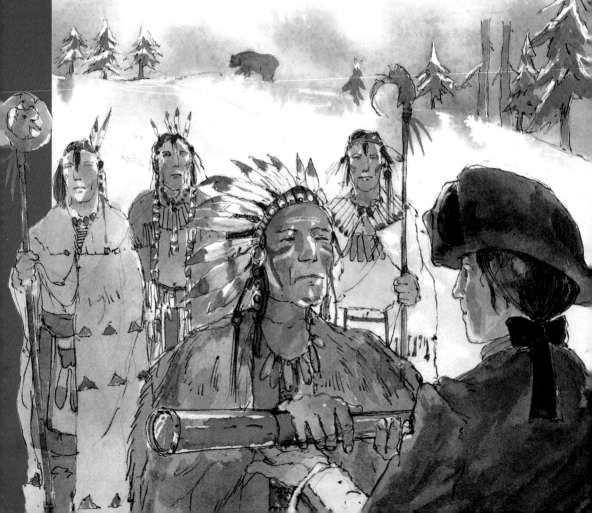

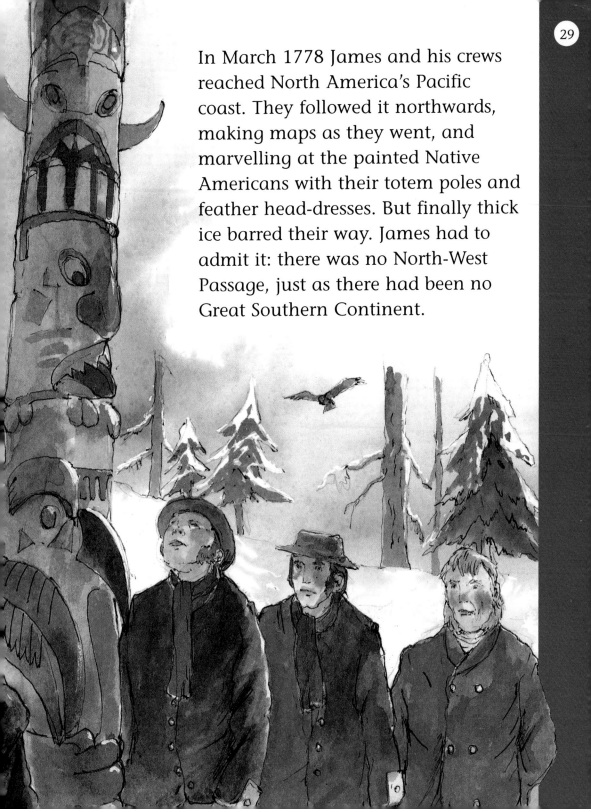

In March 1778 James and his crews reached North America's Pacific coast. They followed it northwards, making maps as they went, and marvelling at the painted Native Americans with their totem poles and feather head-dresses. But finally thick ice barred their way. James had to admit it: there was no North-West Passage, just as there had been no Great Southern Continent.

The *Resolution* and *Discovery* now had to turn and head back south. James remembered how friendly the people of Hawaii had been. He decided to call there again. The two ships arrived in January 1779.

But this time the Hawaiians were in a different mood. They kept picking quarrels with the crews and stealing their belongings. James was furious. On 14 February he tried to sort out the trouble on his own, at Kealakekua Bay. The Hawaiians were confused. They panicked, surrounded James, then attacked him. When they stepped away, Captain Cook was dead.

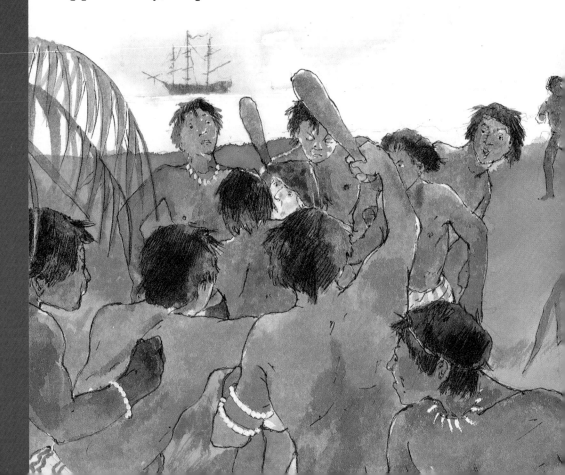

James once wrote that he wanted "to go as far as it is possible for man to go". On his three great voyages of exploration, he went further than any other man of his time. He helped to complete the map of the world.

Today there are still places named after him in Alaska, Australia, New Zealand and Polynesia.

Cook
Inlet

PACIFIC
OCEAN

Cook
Islands

Cook
Strait

Mount
Cook

# Important dates in Captain Cook's life

**1728** James Cook born in Marton, England.

**1746** James becomes a ship's boy on a coal ship.

**1755** James leaves the coal ships to join the Royal Navy.

**1759** James's charts of the St Lawrence River help win the battle for Quebec.

**1762** James marries Elizabeth Batts.

**1768–70** On his first major voyage, James visits Tahiti and charts coasts of New Zealand and Australia.

**1772–75** On his second voyage, James sights Antarctica and tests the chronometer.

**1776–79** James's final voyage, to look for a north-west passage around America.

**1779** James killed by angry Hawaiians in Kealakekua Bay.

# Index